Current Clinical Strategies

Pediatrics

1995 Edition

Paul D. Chan, M.D.

Edited By

Donald E. Maldonado, M.D.

Preface

Current Clinical Strategies provides a link between the current pediatric literature and the hospital wards. For each disease entity covered, the special nursing orders, diagnostic tests, and therapeutic alternatives are presented. It is the most current source for therapeutic strategies available, including up-to-the-minute information on the treatment of AIDS and other modern diseases. This reference provides help for physicians and medical students who would like to write comprehensive admitting orders; it prevents omission of important laboratory tests and therapeutic measures.

This manual is structured to allow the clinician to individualize patient care by selecting diagnostic tests based upon clinical indications, and then to choose the clinically indicated treatment plan from the alternatives provided. Some of the specific orders may not be appropriate for a given patient, and the physician should use his or her own judgement to select orders as required by the clinical picture.

Publishing information for authors may be obtained by writing to:

Current Clinical Strategies Publishing
9550 Warner Ave, Suite 213
Fountain Valley, CA 92708-2822
Phone: 714-965-9400
Fax: 714-965-9401

Printed in USA   ISBN 1-881528-02-2

CONTENTS

GENERAL PEDIATRICS

PEDIATRICS HISTORY & PHYSICAL

Chief Complaint:
History of Present Illness:
Past Medical History:
Medications:
Feedings:
Immunizations:
Birth History:
Developmental:
Family History:
Social History:
Allergies:
Physical exam:
Weight & Height:
Assessment & Plan:

DEVELOPMENTAL MILESTONES

AGE	MILESTONE
1 mo:	Raises head slightly when prone; alerts to sound; regards face, moves extremities equally.
3 mo:	Smiles; holds head up; coos, reaches for familiar objects, laughs; recognizes parent.
4-5 mo:	Rolls front to back and back to front; sits well when propped. Orients to voice; enjoys looking around surroundings, grasps rattle, bears some weight on legs.
6 mo:	Sits unsupported; stranger anxiety; passes cube hand to hand; babbles; uses raking grasp; feeds self crackers.
9 mo:	Crawls, cruises; pulls to stand; pincer grasp; plays pat-a-cake; understands "no"; says "mama/dada" discriminately; feeds self with bottle; sits without support; explores environment.
12 mo:	Walking; talking a few words; throws objects; comes when called; imitates actions.
15-18 mo:	Scribbles; walks backward; uses 4-20 words; builds tower of 2 blocks; points to body parts; runs; spoon feeds self; copies parents.
24-30 mo:	Removes shoes; follows 2 step command; jumps with both feet; holds pencil; knows first & last name; knows pronouns. Parallel

	play.
3 yr:	Dresses & undresses; walks up & down steps; draws a circle; knows more than 250 words; takes turns; shares. Group play.
4 yr:	Hops; skips; catches ball; memorizes songs; plays cooperatively; knows colors.
5 yr:	Jumps over objects; prints first name; ties shoes; knows address & mother's name; tolerates separation; follows game rules.

Note: These milestones are intended for general sequence only. Premature infants must be age corrected for their prematurity prior to testing.

IMMUNIZATION

Recommended Schedule for Immunization of Healthy Infants and Children:

Recommended Age	Immunizations	Comments
Birth	HBV	
1-2 mo	HBV	
2 mo	DTP, Hib, OPV	DTP and OPV can be initiated as early as 4 wk in high endemicity areas
4 mo	DTP, Hib, OPV	2-mo interval (minimum 6 wk) for OPV
6 mo	DTP, (Hib)	Dose 3 of Hib is not indicated if the product for doses 1 and 2 was PedvaxHIB.
6-18 mo	HBV, OPV	
12-15 mo	Hib, MMR	Tuberculin testing may be done at the same visit
15-18 mo	DTaP or DTP	The 4th dose of DTP should be given 6-12 mo after third dose of DTP and may be given as early as 12 mo, provided that the interval between doses 3 and 4 is at least 6 mo
4-6 y	DTaP or DTP, OPV	DTaP or DTP and OPV should be given at or before school entry. DTP or DTaP should not be given at or after the 7th birthday
11-12 y	MMR	MMR should be given at entry to middle school or junior high school
14-16 y	Td	Repeat every 10 yrs throughout life

HBV = Hepatitis B virus vaccine; DTP = diphtheria and tetanus toxoids and pertussis vaccine; DTaP = diphtheria and tetanus toxoids and acellular pertussis vaccine; Hib = Haemophilus influenzae type b conjugate vaccine; OPV = oral poliovirus vaccine (attenuated); MMR = live measles, mumps, and rubella viruses vaccine; Td = adult tetanus toxoid (full dose) and diphtheria toxoid (reduced dose), for children >7 y and adults.

HAEMOPHILUS IMMUNIZATION

Recommendations for H influenzae type b Vaccination in Children Immunized Beginning at 2 to 6 Months of Age

Vaccine Product at Initiation	Total Number of Doses to Be Administered	Currently Recommended Vaccine Regimens
HbOC or PRP-T	4	3 doses at 2-mo intervals Same vaccine for doses 1-3 Fourth dose at 12 to 15 mo of age Any conjugate vaccine for dose 4
PRP-OMP	3	2 doses at 2-mo intervals Same vaccine for doses 1 and 2 Third dose at 12-15 mo of age Any conjugate vaccine for dose 3

Recommendations for H influenzae type b Vaccination in Children in Whom Initial Vaccination was Delayed Until 7 Months of Age or Older

Age at Initiation of Immunization	Vaccine Product	Total Number of Doses to Be Administered	Currently Recommended Vaccine Regimens
7-11 mo	HbOC, PRP-T, or PRP-OMP	3	2 doses at 2-mo intervals Same vaccine for doses 1 and 2 Third dose at 12-18 mo, given at least 2 mo after dose 2 Any conjugate vaccine for dose 3
12-14 mo	HbOC, PRP-T, PRP-D	2	2-mo interval between doses Any conjugate vaccine for dose 2
15-59	HbOC, PRP-T, PRP-OMP, or PRP-D	1	Any conjugate vaccine
60 and older	HbOC, PRP-T, PRP-OMP, or PRP-D	1 or 2	Any conjugate vaccine; only for children with chronic illness at increased risk for H influenzae type b disease

PEDIATRIC SYMPTOMATIC CARE

FEVER

Definition of Fever:

Rectal Temperature	>38 degrees Celsius
Oral Temperature	>37.5 degrees Celsius
Axillary Temperature	>37 degrees Celsius

Analgesics:

-Acetaminophen (Tylenol) 10-20 mg/kg/dose q4-6h PO/PR, max 5 doses/d **OR**

-Acetaminophen dose by age (if weight appropriate for age):

AGE:	**Mg/Dose PO q4-6h:**
0-3 mo	40 mg/dose
4-11 mo	80 mg/dose
1-2 yr	120 mg/dose
2-3 yr	160 mg/dose
4-5 yr	240 mg/dose
6-8 yr	320 mg/dose
9-10 yr	400 mg/dose
11-12 yr	480 mg/dose
>12 yr	325-650 mg q4h

-Preparations - 325, 500 mg tabs; 80 mg chewable tabs; 160 mg caplets; 80 mg/0.8 ml drops; 120/5 ml, 130/5 ml, 160/5 ml, 325 mg/5 ml elixir; 160 mg/5 ml syrup; 120,325,650 mg suppositories. Max dosage 4 grams per 24 hours; Contraindicated in patients with known G6PD deficiency.

-Ibuprofen (Motrin, Advil, Nuprin, Medipren, Children's Motrin), antipyretic: 20 mg/kg/d q8h PO. Max dose: 40 mg/kg/d. [suspension: 100 mg/5 ml, tabs: 200, 300, 400, 600, 800 mg]. May cause GI distress, bleeding.

Other Orders & Meds:

COUGH & CONGESTION

Antitussives (Pure):

-Guaifenesin (Robitussin), expectorant: <2 y: 12 mg/kg/d PO q4-6h prn; 2-5 yr: 50-100 mg q4h, max 600 mg/d; 6-11 yr: 100-200 mg q4h, max 1.2 g/d; >12 yr: 200-400 mg q4h, max 2.4 g/d [100 mg/5 ml syrup]. may irritate gastric mucosa; take with large quantities of fluids.

Decongestants:

-Pseudoephedrine (Sudafed, Novafed): children <12 yr: 4 mg/kg/d divided q6h. Children >12 yr and adults: 30-60 mg/dose q6-8h PO, Sustained

release 120 mg PO q12h. Max dose: 240 mg/24h. [Tabs: 30, 60 mg; sustained release caps: 120 mg; syrup: 15, 30 mg/5 ml; drops: 7.5 mg/0.8 ml]
-PediaCare infant drops (pseudoephedrine 7.5 mg/0.8 ml dropper), 4-5 mg/kg/d PO q6h.

Combinations (Antihistamine/Decongestant/Antitussive):
-Actifed OTC (Triprolidine 2.5 mg, Pseudoephedrine 60 mg per tab or 10 ml syrup) 4 mg pseudoephedrine/kg/d PO tid-qid. 4 mth-2 y: 1.25 ml q6-8h; 2-4 y: 2.5 ml q6-8h; 4-6 y: 3.75 ml q6-8h; 6-12y: 5 ml q6-8h; >12 y: 10 ml q6-8h.
-Actifed with Codeine cough syrup (Codeine 10 mg, Triprolidine 1.25 mg, Pseudoephedrine 30 mg/5 ml) 4 mg pseudoephedrine/kg/d PO tid-qid. 4 mth-2 y: 1.25 ml q6-8h; 2-4 y: 2.5 ml q6-8h; 4-6 y: 3.75 ml q6-8h; 6-12y: 5 ml q6-8h; >12 y: 10 ml q6-8h.
-Benylin DM Cough Syrup (Dextromethorphan 10 mg/5 ml) 2-5 y: 2.5-5 mg q4h PO or 7.5 mg q6-8h; 6-11 y 5-10 mg q4h or 15 mg q6-8h; ≥12 y: 10-20 mg q4h or 30 mg q6-8h.
-Dimetapp (Brompheniramine 2 mg/Phenylpropanolamine 12.5 mg/5 ml) 1-6 mth: 1.25 ml PO q6-8h; 7-24 m: 2.5 ml q6-8h; 2-4 y: 3.75 ml q6-8h; 4-11 y: 5 ml q6-8h; or ≥12 y: 5-10 ml q6-8h or 0.5 mg/kg/d of brompheniramine component q6-8h [4/25 mg tabs; 2/12.5/per 5 ml Elixir; sustained release tab 12/75 mg].
-Dimetane elixir OTC (3% alcohol; brompheniramine 2 mg/5 ml) 0.5 mg/kg/d q6-8h or SR q12h, max 24 mg/d [tab, 4 mg; SR tab, 8,12 mg]
-Entex (Phenylpropanolamine 20 mg/Phenylephrine 5 mg/Guaifenesin 100 mg/5 ml) 6-12 yrs: 5 ml qid; or ≥ 12 yr: Entex LA 1 tab bid [scored tab 75/0/400 mg].
-PediaCare I Children's Cough Relief Liquid (Dextromethorphan 5 mg/5 ml) 2-5 y: 2.5-5 mg q4h or 7.5 mg q6-8h; 6-11 y 5-10 mg q4h or 15 mg q6-8h; ≥12 y: 10-20 mg q4h or 30 mg q6-8h.
-PediaCare 3 Children's Cold Relief Liquid (Dextromethorphan 5 mg, chlorpheniramine 1 mg, pseudoephedrine 15 mg/5 ml) dose as per pseudoephedrine component: 4-5 mg/kg/d q6h.
-Phenergan VC with Codeine (Promethazine 6.25 mg, Codeine 10 mg, phenylephrine 5 mg/5 ml) 2-6 yrs 1.25 ml/dose or 6-12 yrs: 2.5-5 ml/dose q4-6h or >12 yrs 5 ml q4-6h.
-Phenergan with Dextromethorphan (Promethazine 6.25 mg, Dextromethorphan 15 mg/5 ml) 2-5 y: 2.5-5 mg q4h or 7.5 mg q6-8h; 6-11 y 5-10 mg q4h or 15 mg q6-8h; ≥12 y: 10-20 mg q4h or 30 mg q6-8h.
-Robitussin AC (Guaifenesin 100 mg, Codeine, 10 mg per 5 ml), 2-6 yrs: 2.5 ml q4h; 6-12 yrs: 5 ml q4h; ≥12 yrs: 10 ml q4-6h.
-Robitussin CF (Guaifenesin 100 mg, Dextromethorphan 10 mg, Phenylpropanolamine 12.5 mg per 5 ml), 2-6 yrs: 2.5 ml q4h; 6-12 yrs: 5 ml q4h; ≥12 yrs: 10 ml q4-6h..

- Robitussin DM (Guaifenesin 100 mg, Dextromethorphan 15 mg/5 ml) dose as per guaifenesin component: 2-6 y: 50-100 mg q4h, max 600 mg/d; 6-11 y: 100-200 mg, max 1200 mg/d; ≥12 y: 200-400 mg q4h, max 2.4 g/d.
- Rondec syrup (Pseudoephedrine 60 mg, carbinoxamine 4 mg/5 ml) dose per pseudoephedrine: 4-5 mg/kg/d q6h.
- Rondec DM drops (carbinoxamine maleate 2 mg, pseudoephedrine 25 mg, dextromethorphan 4 mg/ml) dose per pseudoephedrine: 4-5 mg/kg/d q6h; or 1-3 m: ¼ dropperful (¼ ml) q6h; 3-6 m: ½ dropperful q6h; 6-9 m: 3/4 dropperful q6h; 9-18 m: 1 dropperful q6h.
- Rondec drops (carbinoxamine maleate 2 mg, pseudoephedrine 25 mg/ml), same dose as Rondec DM drops.
- Sudafed Cough Syrup (Dextromethorphan 5 mg, guaifenesin 100 mg, pseudoephedrine 15 mg/5 ml) dose per pseudoephedrine: 4-5 mg/kg/d q6h.
- Sudafed plus (Pseudoephedrine 30 mg, chlorpheniramine 2 mg/5 ml) dose per pseudoephedrine: 4-5 mg/kg/d q6h.
- Tavist-D (Tabs: Clemastine 1.34 mg, Phenylpropanolamine 75 mg) ≥ 12 y: 1 tab bid [SR tab].
- Triaminic Expectorant (Yellow) (phenylpropanolamine 12.5/5 ml, guaifenesin 100 mg/5 ml), 3-12 mth: 0.75 ml (1/8 tsp) q4h; 12-24 mth: 1.25 ml (¼ tsp) q4-8h; 2-6 y: 2.5 ml (½ tsp) q4-8h.
- Triaminic syrup (phenylpropanolamine 12.5, chlorpheniramine 2 mg/ 5 ml), 3-12 months 12: 0.75 ml (1/8 tsp) q4h; 12-24 mth: 1.25 ml (¼ tsp) q4-8h; 2-6 yrs: 2.5 ml (½ tsp) q4h.
- Triaminic-DM (phenylpropanolamine 12.5, dextromethorphan 10 mg/5 ml), same dose as Triaminic syrup.
- Triaminicol (phenylpropanolamine 12.5, chlorpheniramine 2 mg, dextromethorphan 10 mg/5 ml), 3-12 mth: 0.75 ml (1/8 tsp) q4h; 12-24 mth: 1.25 ml (¼ tsp) q4h; 2-5 y: 2.5 ml q4h; 6-11 y: 5 ml q4h.
- Phenylephrine nasal drops (Neo-Synephrine) 1/8, ¼, ½, 1%; or nasal spray: ¼, ½, 1%; infants 1/8 % drops, 1-2 drops each nostril q3-4h; children: ¼ % spray or drops, 1-2 drops/spray q3-4h; adults ¼-1% drops/spray 1-2 drops/sprays q3-4h; discontinue use after 3 days to avoid rebound congestion.

PAIN & SEDATION

Pain:

- Acetaminophen/Codeine 0.5-1.0 mg codeine/kg/dose PO q4h prn [Acetaminophen 120 mg & Codeine 12 mg/5 ml; or tabs Tylenol #2: 15 mg codeine/300 mg acetaminophen; #3: 30/300 mg; #4: 60/300 mg].
- Acetaminophen (Tylenol) 10-15 mg/kg PO q4-6h (see page 10) **OR**
- Morphine 0.08-0.1 mg/kg IV q2-4h prn or 0.02-0.06 mg/kg/h IV infusion; or 0.1-0.15 mg/kg IM/SC q3-4h

-Meperidine (Demerol) 1 mg/kg IV/IM q2-3h prn.
-Fentanyl 1-2 mcg/kg IV q1-2h prn or 1-2 mcg/kg/h continuous IV infusion.
-Hydromorphone (Dilaudid) 0.015-0.03 mg/kg IV/IM/SC q3-4h
-Methadone 0.1-0.2 mg/kg PO/IV q6-12h.
-Ibuprofen (Children's Motrin, PediaProfen) >6 mth: 5-10 mg/kg/dose PO q6-8h [100 mg/5 ml; tabs 200,300,400,600,800 mg]
-EMLA cream (eutectic mixture of local anesthetics) 2.5% lidocaine and 2.5% prilocaine, Apply at least 1 hour prior to procedure (lumbar puncture, venipuncture, marrow aspiration).

Sedation:
DPT Cocktail (may mix in same syringe):
-Meperidine (Demerol) 1-2 mg/kg IM **AND**
-Promethazine (Phenergan) 0.5-1 mg/kg IM **AND**
-Chlorpromazine (Thorazine) 0.5-1 mg/kg IM.
Fentanyl & Midazolam Sedation:
-Fentanyl, 1-3 years: 2-3 mg/kg/dose; 3-12 years: 1-2 mg/kg/dose **AND**
-Midazolam (Versed) 0.05-0.1 mg/kg slow IV [inj 1 mg/ml, 5 mg/ml].
Other Sedatives (one time agents, pre-procedure):
-Lorazepam (Ativan) 0.05-0.10 mg/kg/dose IM/IV/PO, max 4 mg.
-Diazepam (Valium) 0.2-0.5 mg/kg/dose PO or 0.05-0.2 mg/kg/dose IV, max 10 mg.
-Midazolam (Versed) 0.08-0.15 mg/kg/dose IM/IV over 10-20 min, max 5 mg; or 0.2-0.4 mg/kg/dose PO x 1 (max 15 mg) 30-45 min prior to procedure; or 0.2 mg/kg intranasal.
-Chloral Hydrate 25-100 mg/kg/dose PO, PR (max 1.5 gm/dose), allow 30min for absorption.
-Promethazine (Phenergan) 0.5-1 mg/kg/dose IM or slow IV over 20 min, max 50 mg.
-Chlorpromazine (Thorazine) 0.5-1 mg/kg/dose IM or slow IV over 20min (max 50 mg/dose).
-Hydroxyzine (Vistaril) 0.5-1 mg/kg/dose IM, max 50 mg.

Precautionary Measures:
-Naloxone (Narcan) opiate antagonist 0.1 mg/kg IV/IM (have available to counteract sedation/respiratory depression).
-Flumazenil (Mazicon) 0.01 mg/kg IV (available 0.1 mg/ml in 5 ml and 10 ml vials) (benzodiazepine antagonist)

NAUSEA & VOMITING

-Chlorpromazine (Thorazine) 0.25-0.50 mg/kg/dose, (max 50 mg) IM, slow IV over 20 min or PO q4-6h or 1 mg/kg/dose PR q6-8h [25 mg/ml inj, 10 mg/5 ml oral syrup, 30 mg/ml oral concentrate; 10,25,50,100,200 mg tabs; 25-,100 mg supp].

-Dimenhydrinate (Dramamine) ≥12 yrs: 5 mg/kg/d IM/IV/PO qid, max 300 mg; not recommended in <12y due to high incidence of extrapyramidal side effects [oral liquid 12.5 mg/4 ml; 50 mg tab; 50 mg/ml inj].

-Diphenhydramine (Benadryl) 1 mg/kg/dose IM/IV/PO qid [oral liquid 12.5 mg/5 ml; 25, 50 mg caps; 10, 50 mg/ml inj].

-Prochlorperazine (Compazine) ≥12 yrs: 0.1-0.15 mg/kg/dose IM, max 10 mg x 1 dose; 0.4 mg/kg/d PO q6-8h, max 40 mg/d; not recommended in <12y due to high incidence of extrapyramidal side effects [5, 10, 25 mg tabs; 30 mg/ml oral concentrate; 5 mg/5 ml syrup; 2.5, 5, 25 mg supp; 5 mg/ml inj].

-Promethazine (Phenergan) 0.25-0.5 mg/kg/dose (max 50 mg) PO/IM/IV over 20min or PR q4-6h [12.5, 25, 50 mg tabs; 12.5, 25, 50 mg supp; 25,50 mg/ml inj].

-Trimethobenzamide (Tigan) 15 mg/kg/d IM/PO/PR q6-8h [100, 250 mg caps; 100, 200 mg supp; 100 mg/ml inj].

CARDIOLOGY

PEDIATRIC ADVANCED LIFE SUPPORT

GENERAL MEASURES:
Begin CPR, 100% oxygen, assess rhythm & pulse. Assess airway, breathing, and circulation; consider nasogastric tube if supportive ventilation required for longer than 2 min.

INTUBATION:
Intubation:

Age:	ETT	Laryngoscope Blade
Premie	2.5-3,0	0
Newborn	3,0-3.5	1
Infant	3,5-4.0	1
12 mo	4.0-4.5	1.5
36 mo	4.5-5.0	2
6 yr	5.0-5.5	2
10 yr	6.0-6.5	2
Adolescent	7.0-7.5	3
Adult	7.5-8.0	3

Uncuffed ET tube in children< 8 yrs.
Straight laryngoscope blade if < 6-10 yrs; curved blade if older.
Preoxygenate with 100% oxygen via air bag and mask.

1. **Atropine** 0.01-0.02 mg/kg IV (min 0.1 mg, max 1 mg).
2. **Lorazepam (Ativan)** 0.1 mg/kg IV (max 4 mg) **OR**
3. **Diazepam (Valium)** 0.2-0.5 mg/kg IV (max 10 mg).
4. **Succinylcholine** 1-2 mg/kg IV (max 100 mg) **OR**
5. **Pancuronium (neonates):** 0.06-0.1 mg/kg/dose IV or children 0.1 mg/kg/dose IV.

SUPRAVENTRICULAR TACHYCARDIA:
1. **Mild to Moderate Severity:** Vagal Stimulation: Ice bag to face 15-20 seconds, rectal stimulation. If no conversion, give Adenosine 0.1 mg/kg rapid IV push; if necessary, increase dose by 0.05 mg/kg increments, repeat every 2 minutes prn until termination of SVT (max dose 0.25 mg/kg, max total dose 12 mg).
2. **Severe:** **Synchronized DC cardiovert** with **0.5-1.0 J/kg**. Double if not successful. Proceed to digitalization.
3. **Maintain oxygenation and ventilation.** Also see page 20.

ASYSTOLE:

1. Start CPR & secure IV access; confirm with 2 leads.
2. **Epinephrine** 0.01 mg/kg (0.1 ml/kg; 0.1 mg/ml = 1:10,000) IV/IM/IO q5min, then 0.05-1 mcg/kg/min continuous IV infusion. Endotracheal High dose epinephrine 0.1 mg/kg (1:1,000 = 1 mg/cc) or 0.1 cc/kg q5min.
3. **Atropine** 0.02 mg/kg (0.2 ml/kg; 1:10,000 sln = 0.1 mg/ml) IV/IM/IO/ET q5min; minimum 0.1 mg/dose, max 1 mg/dose.
4. Consider **External or Transvenous Pacing** & consider **Bicarbonate** for suspected or proven acidosis, 1 mEq/kg IV/IO [1 mEq/ml sln diluted 1:1 with D5W/NS]; in newborns give 2 cc/kg of 0.5 mEq/cc soln.

SINUS BRADYCARDIA:

1. **Atropine** 0.02 mg/kg (0.2 ml/kg; 1:10,000 sln = 0.1 mg/ml) IV/IM/IO/ET q5min; minimum 0.1 mg/dose, max 1 mg/dose.
2. **Isoproterenol** 0.1-1.5 mcg/kg/min; begin with 0.1 mcg/kg/min and increase every 5-10 min by 0.1 mcg/kg/min until desired effect, tachycardia > 180 bpm, or arrhythmia occurs. Max dose: 2 mcg/kg/min. For use in bradycardia due to heart block only **OR**
3. **Epinephrine** 0.01 mg/kg (0.1 ml/kg; 0.1 mg/ml = 1:10,000) IV/IM/IO q5min, then 0.05-1 mcg/kg/min continuous IV infusion. Endotracheal High dose epinephrine 0.1 mg/kg (1:1,000 = 1 mg/cc) or 0.1 cc/kg q5min.
4. Consider **External or Transvenous Pacing**.

COMPLETE HEART BLOCK:

1. **Isoproterenol** 0.1-1.5 mcg/kg/min; begin with 0.1 mcg/kg/min and increase every 5-10 min by 0.1 mcg/kg/min until desired effect, tachycardia > 180 bpm, or arrhythmia occurs. Max dose: 2 mcg/kg/min. For use in bradycardia due to heart block only **OR**
2. **Atropine** 0.01-0.02 mg/kg (0.2 ml/kg; 1:10000 sln = 0.1 mg/ml) IV/IM/IO/ET q5min; minimum 0.1 mg/dose, max 1 mg/dose.
3. Consider **Transvenous ventricular pacing**.

VENTRICULAR FIBRILLATION or PULSELESS VENTRICULAR TACH:

1. Defibrillate with **unsynchronized 2 Joules/kg** may double & repeat.
2. **Epinephrine** 0.01 mg/kg (0.1 ml/kg; 0.1 mg/ml = 1:10,000) IV/IM/IO/ET q5min, then 0.05-1 mcg/kg/min continuous IV infusion. High dose epineph-rine 0.1 mg/kg (1:1,000 = 1 mg/cc) q5min.
3. **Intubate and Ventilate**.
4. **Defibrillate at double previous energy or 3-5 J/kg**, max 360 J.
5. **Lidocaine** 1 mg/kg IV/IO bolus, then 10-50 mcg/kg/min, or dilute in 10 ml of NS via ET tube. **Defibrillate**.
6. **Bretylium tosylate** 5 mg/kg IV/IO bolus (max 500 mg), followed by doses of 10 mg/kg q15-30 min, to max total of 30 mg/kg.
7. **Consider bicarbonate**, 1 mEq/kg IV/IO. **Defibrillate**.

8. **Repeat Bretylium** 10 mg/kg IV bolus q5-10 min until max of 30 mg/kg given. Repeat **Defibrillation**.

9. **Repeat Bretylium or Defibrillation**. Consider **Procainamide** 3-6 mg/kg slow IV over 5min, max 100 mg/dose.

UNSTABLE V TACH WITH PULSE (chest pain, dyspnea, MI, systolic <90, CHF):

1. IV; consider **Midazolam*** (Versed) 0.1 mg/kg IV sedation.

2. Cardiovert with **Synchronized* 12 Joules/kg**, may double and repeat.

3. **Lidocaine** 1 mg/kg IV bolus (max 100 mg), then 20-50 mcg/kg/min IV.

4. If no conversion, **Cardiovert Synchronized*** at double previous rate, or if **recurrent V tach**, **Cardiovert** again starting at previously successful energy level.

5. **Procainamide*** 3-6 mg/kg IV over 5min until conversion or max 15 mg/kg or 100 mg/dose; infusion: 20-80 mcg/kg/min.

6. **Bretylium** 5 mg/kg (max 500 mg) rapid IV over 1-2min, may double & repeat in 20min.

*If unconscious, pulmonary edema, hypotensive, use unsynchronized cardioversion and bypass sedation & procainamide.

STABLE V TACH WITH PULSE:

1. **Lidocaine** 1 mg/kg (max 100 mg) IV then 20-50 mcg/kg/min IV.

2. **Procainamide** 3-6 mg/kg slow IV, may repeat to max 15 mg/kg or 100 mg; infusion: 20-80 mcg/kg/min IV.

3. **Propranolol** 0.01-0.10 mg/kg/dose (max 1 mg) slow IV push **OR Phenytoin** 2-4 mg/kg IV over 5min q15min, max total dose 10-15 mg/kg

4. If no conversion, or if chest pain, dyspnea, or MI, use synchronized cardioversion as in unstable ventricular tachycardia.

CONGESTIVE HEART FAILURE

1. **Admit to:**
2. **Diagnosis:** Congestive Heart Failure
3. **Condition:**
4. **Vital signs:** Call MD if:
5. **Activity:**
6. **Nursing:** Daily weights, I&O
7. **Diet:** Low salt diet
8. **IV Fluids:**
9. **Special Medications:**
   -Oxygen 2-4 L/min by NC.
   -Furosemide (Lasix) 1 mg/kg/dose (usual max 80 mg PO, 40 mg IV) IV/IM/PO

q6-12h prn, may increase to 2 mg/kg/dose IV/IM/PO [20, 40, 80 mg tabs; 10 mg/ml inj; 10 mg/ml PO liquid or 40 mg/5 ml oral soln.].

-Bumetanide (Bumex) 0.015 mg/kg PO q12-24h max 10 mg/d [0.5, 1, 2 mg tabs; 0.25 mg/ml inj].

Digoxin:

Before administration: baseline ECG, serum electrolytes (particularly potassium), estimation of renal function

Digoxin Is Administered in Two Stages:

Initial digitalization establishes the body stores, and is given over 24 hours in three divided doses: 1/2 TDD at time 0 hours, 1/4 TDD at 12 hours, and 1/4 TDD at 24 hours.

Maintenance therapy is then administered, which is generally calculated as 1/8 TDD q12h (thus, 1/4 TDD per day).

Approximate total digitalizing doses (reduced 25% if IV):

(1) Premature: 0.020 mg/kg PO

(2) Full-term newborn: 0.030 mg/kg PO

(3) Under 2 years: 0.040 mg/kg PO

(4) Over 2 years: 0.030-0.040 mg/kg PO

(5) Adult: maximum of 1.0 mg total PO

Maintenance dose is 25-35% of oral digitalizing dose, divided bid.

In < 10 yr: digitalizing doses given as 1/2 the total digitalizing dose initially then 1/4 the total digitalizing dose q8-18 hr x 2.

Divide bid if <10 yrs or qd if ≥10 yrs.

[50, 100, 200 mcg caps; 0.125, 0.250, 0.500 mg tabs; 50 mcg/ml elixir; 100 mcg/ml (1 ml) inj, 250 mcg/ml (2 ml) inj].

Other Inotropic Agents:

-Dopamine 2-30 mcg/kg/min continuous IV infusion, and titrate cardiac output and BP **AND/OR**

-Dobutamine 2.5-15 mcg/kg/min continuous IV infusion, max of 40 mcg/kg/min **AND/OR**

-Nitroglycerine 1 mcg/kg/min continuous IV infusion, may increase by 1 mcg/kg q20min; titrated to MAP >70 mm Hg, systolic >90 mm Hg; max 5 mcg/kg/min.

-Captopril (Capoten), neonates: 0.05-0.1 mg/kg/dose PO q6-8h; infants & children: 0.15 mg/kg/dose PO q8h, max 6 mg/kg/d [tabs 12.5,25,50,100 mg]

-KCL 1-4 mEq/kg/d PO qd.

10. Extras & X-rays: CXR PA & LAT, ECG, echocardiogram.

11. Labs: ABG, SMA 7, CBC, cardiac enzymes, iron studies. Digoxin level at least 8h after dose, UA.

12. Other orders and meds:

ATRIAL FIBRILLATION & ATRIAL FLUTTER

1. **Admit to:**
2. **Diagnosis:** Atrial fibrillation / flutter
3. **Condition:**
4. **Vital signs:** Call MD if:
5. **Activity:**
6. **Nursing:**
7. **Diet:**
8. **IV Fluids:**
9. **Special Medications:**

Cardioversion (if unstable or refractory to drug Tx):

1. If unstable, **Synchronized Cardiovert** immediately. In stable patient, consider starting quinidine or procainamide 24-48h prior.
2. Midazolam (Versed) 0.1 mg/kg IV over 2 min repeat prn until amnesic.
3. Synchronous cardioversion: 0.25-1 Joules/kg. Consider esophageal overdrive pacing.

Rate Control:

Digoxin:

Before administration: baseline ECG, serum electrolytes (particularly potassium), estimation of renal function

Digoxin Is Administered in Two Stages:

Initial digitalization establishes the body stores, and is given over 24 hours in three divided doses: 1/2 TDD at time 0 hours, 1/4 TDD at 12 hours, and 1/4 TDD at 24 hours.

Maintenance therapy is then administered, which is generally calculated as 1/8 TDD q12h (thus, 1/4 TDD per day).

Approximate total digitalizing doses (reduced 25% if IV):

(1) Premature: 0.020 mg/kg PO
(2) Full-term newborn: 0.030 mg/kg PO
(3) Under 2 years: 0.040 mg/kg PO
(4) Over 2 years: 0.030-0.040 mg/kg PO
(5) Adult: maximum of 1.0 mg total PO

Maintenance dose is 25-35% of oral digitalizing dose, divided bid.

In < 10 yr: digitalizing doses given as 1/2 the total digitalizing dose initially then 1/4 the total digitalizing dose q8-18 hr x 2.

Divide bid if <10 yrs or qd if ≥10 yrs.

[50, 100, 200 mcg caps; 0.125, 0.250, 0.500 mg tabs; 50 mcg/ml elixir; 100 mcg/ml (1 ml) inj, 250 mcg/ml (2 ml) inj]. **OR**

Other Rate Controlling Agents:

-Propranolol 0.01-0.1 mg/kg IV, repeat q6-8h prn (max 1 mg/dose). or 0.5-4 mg/kg/d PO q6-8h (max 60 mg/d)[tabs 10,20,40,60,80,90 mg; inj 1 mg/ml; oral solutions: 4 mg/ml, 8 mg/ml].

Pharmacologic Conversion (after rate control):

-Procainamide loading dose of 2-6 mg/kg/dose IV over 5 min, then 20-80 mcg/-kg/min IV infusion (max 100 mg/dose or 2 gm/24h). Then 15-50 mg/kg/d PO q3-6h (max 4 gm/d).

10. Extras & X-rays: Portable CXR, ECG 24h Holter; echocardiogram.

11. Labs: CBC, SMA 7, UA, ABG. Serum drug levels.

12.   Other Orders and Meds:

PAROXYSMAL SUPRAVENTRICULAR TACHYCARDIA

1. **Admit to:**
2. **Diagnosis:** PSVT
3. **Condition:**
4. **Vital signs:** Call MD if:
5. **Activity:**
6. **Nursing:** ECG monitoring.
7. **Diet:**
8. **IV Fluids:**
9. **Special Medications:**

Also see Advanced Pediatric Life Support, page 15.

Attempt vagal maneuvers, Valsalva, carotid massage, gag reflex before drug therapy.

Cardioversion (if unstable or refractory to drug Tx):

1. Midazolam (Versed) 0.1 mg/kg IV over 2 min repeat prn until amnesic.
2. Synchronous cardioversion 0.25-1 Joules/kg.   Consider esophageal overdrive pacing.

Pharmacologic Therapy

-Adenosine 50-100 mcg/kg/dose rapid IV bolus over 1-2 seconds, followed by saline flush; may repeat within 2 minutes, 75-200 mcg/kg/dose (max total dose 12 mg) **OR**

Digoxin:

Before administration: baseline ECG, serum electrolytes (particularly potassium), estimation of renal function

Digoxin Is Administered in Two Stages:

Initial digitalization establishes the body stores, and is given over 24 hours in three divided doses: 1/2 TDD at time 0 hours, 1/4 TDD at 12 hours, and 1/4 TDD at 24 hours.

Maintenance therapy is then administered, which is generally calculated as 1/8 TDD q12h (thus, 1/4 TDD per day).

Approximate total digitalizing doses (reduced 25% if IV):

(1) Premature: 0.020 mg/kg PO

(2) Full-term newborn: 0.030 mg/kg PO

(3) Under 2 years: 0.040 mg/kg PO

(4) Over 2 years: 0.030-0.040 mg/kg PO

(5) Adult: maximum of 1.0 mg total PO

Maintenance dose is 25-35% of oral digitalizing dose, divided bid.

In < 10 yr: digitalizing doses given as 1/2 the total digitalizing dose initially then 1/4 the total digitalizing dose q8-18 hr x 2.

Divide bid if <10 yrs or qd if ≥10 yrs.

[50, 100, 200 mcg caps; 0.125, 0.250, 0.500 mg tabs; 50 mcg/ml elixir; 100 mcg/ml (1 ml) inj, 250 mcg/ml (2 ml) inj]. **OR**

Other Agents:

-Propranolol 0.01-0.1 mg/kg IV, repeat q6-8h prn (max 1 mg/dose).

-Esmolol hydrochloride (Brevibloc) 500 mcg/kg IV over 1 min, then 50 mcg/kg/min IV infusion, increase by 50 mcg/kg/min q5-10min (max of 300 mcg/kg/min).

10. Extras & X-rays: Portable CXR, ECG.

11. Labs: CBC, SMA 7 & 12, Mg, UA. ABG, TFT's. Drug levels

12. Other Orders and Meds:

WOLF-PARKINSON-WHITE SYNDROME
(re-entry tachycardia)

1. Admit to:

2. Diagnosis: Wolf-Parkinson-White syndrome

3. Condition:

4. Vital signs: Call MD if:

5. Activity:

6. Nursing: ECG monitoring

7. Diet:

8. IV Fluids:

9. Special Medications:

Attempt vagal maneuvers: Valsalva, carotid massage before drug Tx. If unstable or refractory to drug Tx, cardiovert with 1-2 Joules/kg.

-Adenosine 50-100 mcg/kg/dose rapid IV bolus over 1-2 seconds, followed by saline flush; may repeat within 2 minutes, 75-200 mcg/kg/dose (max total dose 12 mg) **OR**

Digoxin:

Before administration: baseline ECG, serum electrolytes (particularly potassium), estimation of renal function

Digoxin Is Administered in Two Stages:

Initial digitalization establishes the body stores, and is given over 24 hours in three divided doses: 1/2 TDD at time 0 hours, 1/4 TDD at 12 hours, and 1/4 TDD at 24 hours.

Maintenance therapy is then administered, which is generally calculated as 1/8 TDD q12h (thus, 1/4 TDD per day).

Approximate total digitalizing doses (reduced 25% if IV):

(1) Premature: 0.020 mg/kg PO

(2) Full-term newborn: 0.030 mg/kg PO

(3) Under 2 years: 0.040 mg/kg PO

(4) Over 2 years: 0.030-0.040 mg/kg PO

(5) Adult: maximum of 1.0 mg total PO

Maintenance dose is 25-35% of oral digitalizing dose, divided bid.

In < 10 yr: digitalizing doses given as 1/2 the total digitalizing dose initially then 1/4 the total digitalizing dose q8-18 hr x 2.

    Divide bid if <10 yrs or qd if ≥10 yrs.

    [50, 100, 200 mcg caps; 0.125, 0.250, 0.500 mg tabs; 50 mcg/ml elixir; 100 mcg/ml (1 ml) inj; 250 mcg/ml (2 ml) inj]. **OR**

-Propranolol 0.01-0.1 mg/kg IV, repeat q6-8h prn (max 1 mg/dose).

10. Extras & X-rays: CXR, ECG, 24h Holter; echocardiogram.

11. Labs: CBC, SMA 7, UA, ABG. Serum drug levels.

12. Other Orders and Meds:

HYPERTENSIVE CRISIS

1. Admit to:

2. Diagnosis: Hypertensive Crisis

3. Condition:

4. Vital signs: Call MD if:

5. Activity:

6. Nursing: ECG, daily weights, I&O.

7. Diet:

8. IV Fluids:

9. Special Medications:

-Nifedipine (Procardia, Adalat) 0.25-0.5 mg/kg (max 10 mg) SL or PO repeat q1-3h prn. <u>Warning:</u> Do not use generic products as concentration of drug within the capsule can vary [10,20 mg capsules].

-Nitroprusside (Nipride) 0.5-8 mcg/kg/min continuous IV infusion titrate to blood pressure.

-Labetalol (Trandate) 0.2 mg/kg (max 20 mg) IV over 2 min or 0.4-1 mg/kg/hr continuous infusion.

-Hydralazine (Apresoline) 0.2-0.8 mg/kg/dose slow IV q2-6h

-Enalaprilat 5-10 mcg/kg/dose IV.

-Phentolamine (pheochromocytoma), 0.05-0.1 mg/kg/dose IV q5min prn, max 5 mg/dose.

10. **Extras & X-rays:** CXR, ECG, CT, renal Doppler & ultrasound, abdominal flat plate.

11. **Labs:** CBC, platelets, SMA 7, BUN, creatinine, ESR; fresh urine for UA with micro now & in 6h. Urine specific gravity, thyroid panel, 24h urine for vanillylmandelic acid, metanephrine, catecholamines, sodium; ANA, complement, ASO titer; toxicology screen.

12. **Other Orders and Meds:**

PULMONOLOGY

ASTHMA

1. **Admit to:**
2. **Diagnosis:** Exacerbation of asthma
3. **Condition:**
4. **Vital signs:** Call MD if:
5. **Activity:**
6. **Nursing:** Pulse oximeter, measure peak flow rate for older patients; ABG prn.
7. **Diet:**
8. **IV Fluids:** D5¼ NS or D5 1/2 NS at 1-1.5 x maintenance.
9. **Special Medications:**
    -Oxygen humidified, 1-6 L/min by NC or 25-80% by mask, keep sat >92%. or >95% for patients with bronchopulmonary dysplasia.

Nebulized Beta 2 Agonists:
    -Albuterol (Ventolin) (0.5%, 5 mg/cc sln) nebulized 0.25-0.5 ml in 2 cc NS q2-6h & prn (ie. 0.2 cc in 2 cc NS); may also be given by continuous aerosol.
    -Terbutaline (Brethine) (1.0%, 10 mg/ml) nebulized 0.2-0.3 mg/kg; max 10 mg in 2 cc NS q1-2h prn or nebulized continuously.

Corticosteroids:
    -Methylprednisolone (Solu-Medrol) 2 mg/kg/dose IV q6h x 4 doses, then 1 mg/kg IV q6h x 3-5 days **OR**
    -Prednisolone (Pediapred) 1-2 mg/kg/day PO x 3-5 days [5 mg/5 ml, 15 mg/5 ml] **OR**
    -Prednisone 1-2 mg/kg/day PO x 3-5 days [1,2.5,5,10,20,50 mg tab; 1 mg/ml, 5 mg/ oral solution].

Anticholinergics:
    -Atropine sulfate (0.5%, 5 mg/ml) 0.05-0.075 mg/kg (max 5 mg) in 2.5 ml NS nebulized (mixed with beta agonist) q6-8h prn; use is limited because of side effects (drying of the oropharynx, increased heart rate, sedation, blurred vision) **OR**
    -Ipratropium Bromide (Atrovent) MDI , <12 yr: 1-2 puffs q6-8h; > 12 yr: 2-4 puffs q6h up to 12 puffs/24h. Fewer side effects and a longer duration of action than atropine. Especially helpful with coexisting chronic bronchitis or cough, intolerance to theophylline or beta-2 agonists, and when beta-adrenergic drugs are inadequate.

Aminophylline & Theophylline:
    -Infrequently used; must follow theophylline levels (10-20 mg/L). Caution advised when given with erythromycin or carbamazepine (Tegretol).
    -Aminophylline loading dose, 5-6 mg/kg **total** body weight in D5¼ NS IV over 20-30 min. 1 mg/kg of aminophylline will raise levels by 2 mg/L.

-Aminophylline maintenance, continuous IV infusion (in D5¼ NS):

    1-6 mth: 0.5 mg/kg/h

    6-12 mth: 0.6-0.75 mg/kg/h

    12 mth-10 y: 1.0 mg/kg/h

    10-16 y: 0.75-0.9 mg/kg/h **OR**

-Theophylline PO loading dose of 6 mg/kg, then maintenance of 80% of total daily maintenance IV aminophylline dose (see above) in 2-4 doses/d (depending on product).

    1-6 mth: 9.6 mg/kg/d theophylline.

    6-12 mth: 11.5-14.4 mg/kg/d theophylline.

    12 mth-10 y: 19.2 mg/kg/d theophylline.

    10-16 y: 14.4-17.3 mg/kg/d theophylline.

-Give theophylline as sustained release theophylline preparation: q8-12h or Liquid immediate Release: q6h.

-Slo-Phyllin Gyrocaps, may open caps & sprinkle on food [60,125,250 mg caps] q8-12h or Slo-Phyllin [100,200 mg] q8-12h **OR**

-Slobid Gyrocaps, may open caps & sprinkle on food [50,75,100,125,200,300 mg caps] q8-12h.

-Theo-Dur [100,200,300,450 mg tabs; scored, may cut in half, but do not crush].

Parenteral Beta Agonists:

-Epinephrine (1 mg/ml, 1:1000) 0.01 ml/kg (0.01 mg/kg)(max 0.5 mg/dose) SQ q15-20min up to 3 doses **OR**

-Albuterol IV solution (Canada only; not FDA approved in US), 1 mcg/kg/min x 10min (loading dose), then 0.2 mcg/kg/min, increase by 0.1 mcg/kg/min increments to max 4 mcg/kg/min.

Beta 2 Agonist, Corticosteroid & Cromolyn Metered Dose Inhalers:

-Albuterol (Ventolin, Proventil) or Metaproterenol (Alupent) MDI 2 puffs q1-6h with spacer & mask.

-Beclomethasone (Beclovent) MDI 1-2 puffs qid or 4 puffs bid (max 16 puffs/d) with spacer & mask, 5 min after bronchodilator, followed by gargling with water **OR**

-Triamcinolone (Azmacort) MDI 1-2 puffs qid or 4 puffs bid (max 16 puffs/d) **OR**

-Flunisolide (AeroBid) MDI 1-2 puffs bid-qid (max 8 puffs/d).

-Cromolyn sodium (Intal) MDI 2-4 puffs qid-tid; or powder 20 mg/capsule bid-qid; or nebulized 1% sln, 1 amp (2 ml, 20 mg) q6h. Not recommended for acute treatment since duration of onset is 2-4 weeks.

Oral Beta 2 Agonists:

-Albuterol liquid (Proventil) 0.1-0.2 mg/kg/dose (max 2 mg if <12 yr; max 4 mg if >12 y) PO q6-8h [2 mg/5 ml or tabs 2 mg, 4 mg] **OR**

-Metaproterenol liquid (Alupent) 0.3-0.5 mg/kg/dose PO q6-8h [10 mg/5 ml; 10 or 20 mg tabs].

11. **Extras & X-rays:** CXR, pulmonary function test, skin allergy testing.

12. Labs: CBC. Theo level. CBG/ABG. Urine antigen screen, UA. Nasopharyngeal washings for direct fluorescent antibody (RSV, adenovirus, parainfluenza, influenza virus, chlamydia) & viral cultures. PPD, sweat test.

13. Other Orders and Meds:

ALLERGIC RHINITIS AND CONJUNCTIVITIS

Antihistamines (also see, cough & rhinorrhea, page 10):
-Actifed OTC (triprolidine 2.5 mg, pseudoephedrine 60 mg per tab or 10 ml syrup) 4 mg pseudoephedrine/kg/d tid-qid. 4 m-2 y: 1.25 ml q6-8h; 2-4 y: 2.5 ml q6-8h; 4-6 y: 3.75 ml q6-8h; 6-12y: 5 ml q6-8h; >12 y: 10 ml q6-8h.

-Chlorpheniramine maleate (Chlor-Trimeton), 0.35 mg/kg/d PO q4-6h [2 mg/5 ml; tabs 4,8,12 mg].

-Hydroxyzine (Vistaril) 2-4 mg/kg/d PO q6h (max 50 mg/dose) [tabs 10, 25, 50,100 mg; susp 5 mg/ml; syrup 2 mg/ml].

-Terfenadine (Seldane), >12 yr: 60 mg PO bid [60 mg tabs]. Cardiac rhythm disturbances have been observed with coadministration of erythromycin. Coadministration with erythromycin is contraindicated.

-Astemizole (Hismanal): 6-12 yr: 5 mg/24 hr PO; >12 yr: 30 mg PO qd x 1 day, then 20 mg PO qd x 1 day, then 10 mg PO qd [10 mg tabs].

Decongestants (also see, cough & rhinorrhea, page 10):
-Pseudoephedrine (Sudafed, Novafed): children <12 yr: 4 mg/kg/d divided q6h. Children >12 yr and adults: 30-60 mg/dose q6-8h PO, Sustained release 120 mg PO q12h. Max dose: 240 mg/24h. [Tabs: 30, 60 mg; sustained release caps: 120 mg; syrup: 15, 30 mg/5 ml; drops: 7.5 mg/0.8 ml]

-Phenylpropanolamine (Tavist) 2-3 mg/kg/d PO q3-4h [liquid].

Intranasal Steroids & Cromolyn:
-Beclomethasone (Beconase) 1-2 sprays each nostril bid-tid. Rinse mouth after use.

-Flunisolide (Nasalide) 1-2 sprays each nostril bid-tid.

-Cromolyn (Nasalcrom) 1 puff in each nostril q3-4h. Not recommended for acute treatment since duration of onset is 2-4 weeks.

Allergic Conjunctivitis Therapy:
-Cromolyn ophthalmic (Opticrom) 2 drops each eye q4-6h.

-Naphazoline/pheniramine (Vasocon A, Opcon A, Naphcon A) 1-2 drops in each eye q4-6h

---

ANAPHYLAXIS

1. **Admit to:**
2. **Diagnosis:** Anaphylaxis
3. **Condition:**
4. **Vital signs:** Call MD if:
5. **Activity:**
6. **Nursing:** I&O. Elevate legs, ECG monitoring.
7. **Diet:**
8. **IV Fluids:** 2 IV lines. Normal saline or LR 10-20 cc/kg rapidly over 1h, then D5½NS at 1-1.5 times maintenance.
9. **Special Medications:**
   -O2 at 6 L/min by NC or mask.
   -Epinephrine, administer 0.01 ml/kg of a 1:1000 concentration (maximum 0.3 ml) subcutaneously and repeat every 15-20 minutes as necessary. If anaphylaxis is the consequence of a sting or intramuscular injection, give a further 0.1 ml of epinephrine at the site to slow antigen absorption. **OR**
   -Epinephrine racemic (stridor) 2% nebulized 0.05 ml/kg/dose in 2.5 cc NS over 15 min q30min-4h (max 0.5 ml/dose).
   -Albuterol (Ventolin) (0.5%, 5 mg/cc sln) nebulized 0.01-0.03 cc/kg (max 1 cc) in 2 cc NS q1-2h & prn; should be used in addition to epinephrine if necessary.

Corticosteroids:
   -Corticosteroids prevent the late phase of the allergic response.
   -If symptoms am mild, give prednisone, initially 2 mg/kg/day (max 40 mg) PO divided q12h, then taper the dose over 4-5 days. For more severe symptoms, give hydrocortisone, 5 mg/kg q8h IV.

Antihistamines:
   -Diphenhydramine (Benadryl) 3-5 mg/kg/day q6h IV/IM/IO/PO q6h, max 50 mg/dose; antihistamines are not a substitute for epinephrine **OR**
   -Hydroxyzine (Vistaril) 1 mg/kg/dose IM/IV/PO q4-6h, max 50 mg/dose

10. **Extras & X-rays:** portable CXR, lateral soft tissue neck x-rays, ECG.
11. **Labs:** CBC, SMA 7, ABG.
12. **Other Orders and Meds:**

PLEURAL EFFUSION

1. **Admit to:**
2. **Diagnosis:** Pleural effusion
3. **Condition:**
4. **Vital signs:** Call MD if:
5. **Activity:**
6. **Diet:**
7. **IV Fluids:**
8. **Extras & X-rays:** CXR PA & LAT, lateral decubitus, ultrasound, ECG, intermediate PPD & candida, mumps skin test. Pulmonary consult.
9. **Labs:** CBC with differential, SMA 7, protein, albumin, amylase, rheumatoid factor, ANA, ESR, UA.

Pleural fluid:

<u>**Tube 1**</u> - LDH, protein, amylase, trig, glucose, specific gravity (10 ml red top).

<u>**Tube 2**</u> - Gram stain, C&S, AFB, fungal C&S, wet mount (20-60 ml).

<u>**Tube 3**</u> - Cell count and differential (5-10 ml, EDTA purple top).

<u>**Tube 4**</u> - Cytology, antigen tests for S pneumoniae, H influenza, rheumatoid factor, (25-50 ml, heparinized).

<u>**Syringe**</u> - pH (2 ml, heparinized).

10. **Other Orders and Meds:**

INFECTIOUS DISEASES

SUSPECTED SEPSIS

1. **Admit to:**
2. **Diagnosis:** Rule out sepsis
3. **Condition:**
4. **Vital signs:** Call MD if:
5. **Activity:**
6. **Nursing:** I&O, daily weights, cooling blanket prn temp > 38°, consent for lumbar puncture. Strict isolation.
7. **Diet:**
8. **IV Fluids:**
9. **Special Medications:**

Term Newborn Infants <1 months old; see "Neonatal Sepsis" page 81.

Infant 1-3 months old (H. flu, pneumococci, meningococci, GpB strep):
  - -Ampicillin, 100 mg/kg/d IV q6h **AND EITHER**
  - -Cefotaxime, 100 mg/kg/d IV q6h **OR**
  - -Ceftriaxone, 50-75 mg/kg/d IV/IM q12-24h.

Children 3 months to 18 years old (S pneumonia, H flu, N. meningitides):
  - -Cefotaxime, 100 mg/kg/d IV q6h, max 12 g/d **OR**
  - -Ceftriaxone, 50-75 mg/kg/d IV/IM q12-24h, max 4 g/d **OR**
  - -Cefuroxime 75-100 mg/kg/d IV q8h, max 9 g/d **OR**
  - -Ceftazidime 100-150 mg/kg/d IV q8h, max 12 gm/d.

Neutropenic Patients (Gram negative, Pseudomonas, Staph, viridans):
  - -Ticarcillin/clavulanate (Timentin) 200-300 mg/kg/d of ticarcillin IV q4-6h, max 18 g/d **OR**
  - -Ceftazidime 100-150 mg/kg/d IV q8h, max 12 gm/d **AND**
  - -Tobramycin or Gentamicin (normal renal function):
    - <5 yr (except neonates): 7.5 mg/kg/d IV q8h.
    - 5-10 yr: 6.0 mg/kg/d IV q8h.
    - >10 yr: 5.0 mg/kg/d IV q8h **AND**
  - -Vancomycin (if patient has central line) 40-60 mg/kg/d IV q6h, max 2 g/d.

10. **Symptomatic Meds:**
  - -Acetaminophen 10-15 mg/kg PO/PR q4-6h prn temp >38° or pain.
11. **Extras & X-rays:** CXR, PPD.
12. **Labs:** CBC, SMA 7. Blood C&S. UA, urine C&S. ESR, antibiotic levels. Stool for wright stain.

Nasopharyngeal washings for direct fluorescent antibody (RSV, adenovirus, parainfluenza, influenza virus, chlamydia) & viral cultures. Urine antigen screen for H flu, group B strep pneumococcus, meningococcus.

  CSF Tube 1 - Gram stain, C&S for bacteria, antigen screen (1-2 ml).

  CSF Tube 2 - Glucose, protein (1-2 ml).

  CSF Tube 3 - Cell count & differential (1-2 ml).

13. Other Orders and Meds:

EMPIRIC THERAPY OF MENINGITIS

1. **Admit to:**
2. **Diagnosis:** Meningitis.
3. **Condition:**
4. **Vital signs:** Call MD if:
5. **Activity:**
6. **Nursing:** Respiratory isolation. I&O, daily weights; cooling blanket prn temp > 38°; consent for lumbar puncture.
7. **Diet:**
8. **IV Fluids:** Isotonic fluids at 2/3 maintenance.
9. **Special Medications:**

Term Newborn Infants <1 months old (Group B strep, E coli, or GpD strep, gram negatives, Listeria):

-Ampicillin, 0-7 d: 200/kg/d IV q12h >7d: 200 mg/kg/d IV q6h **AND**

-Cefotaxime, neonate: <1200 grams: 0-4 wks: 100 mg/kg/d divided q 12 h IV/IM; >1200 grams: 0-7 days: 100 mg/kg/d divided q12h IV/IM; >7 days: 150 mg/kg/d divided q8h IV/IM **OR**

-Ceftriaxone 0-7 d: 50 mg/kg/d IV q24h; >7d: 75 mg/kg/d IV divided q12h or q24h **OR**

-Gentamicin or Tobramycin, 2.5 mg/kg/dose
  Dosing Interval:
  Gestational Age < 28 wks & < 7 days old: q24h; >7 days: q18h
    28-34 wks & < 7 days old: q18h >7 days: q12h
    >34 wks & < 7 days old: q12 h >7 days: q8h

OR

-Amikacin (if gent resistance likely), 7.5 mg/kg/dose IV/IM
  Dosing Interval:
  Gestational Age <28 wks & <7 days old: q24h; >7 days: q18h
    28-34 wks &<7 days old: q18h; >7 days: q 12h
    >34 wks&<7 days old: q12 h; >7 days: q 8h

Infant 1-3 months old (H. flu, pneumococci, meningococci, GpB strep, E coli):

-Ampicillin, 200 mg/kg/d IV q6h **AND EITHER**

-Cefotaxime, 200 mg/kg/d IV q6h **OR**

-Ceftriaxone 100 mg/kg/d IV q12h or qd.

-Dexamethasone 0.15 mg/kg/dose IV q6h x 4 days (16 doses; indicated to decrease inflammation & hearing loss; majority of studies support use in documented H flu infections only).

Children 3 months to 18 years old (S pneumonia, H flu, N. meningitides):
-Cefotaxime, 200 mg/kg/d IV q6h, max 12 g/d **OR**
-Ceftriaxone 100 mg/kg/d IV q12-24h, max 4 g/d **OR**
-Dexamethasone (see above).

10. Symptomatic Meds:
-Acetaminophen 15 mg/kg PO/PR q4h prn temp >38° or pain.

11. Extras & X-rays: CT, CXR, PPD.

12. Labs: CBC, SMA 7. Blood C&S. UA, urine C&S; urine specific gravity. C-reactive protein. Antibiotic levels. Stool for wright stain. Nasopharyngeal washings for direct fluorescent antibody (RSV, adenovirus, parainfluenza, influenza virus, chlamydia) & viral cultures. Urine antigen screen for H flu, group B strep pneumococcus, meningococcus. Throat culture, VDRL; Urine & blood antigen tests.

Lumbar Puncture: (spinal needles, 22 gauge; <1 yrs: 1½ inch, mid-childhood: 2½ inch; adolescents: 3½ inch).

CSF Tube 1 - Gram stain, C&S, bacterial antigen screen (1-2 ml).

CSF Tube 2 - Glucose, protein (1-2 ml).

CSF Tube 3 - Cell count & differential (1-2 ml).

13. Other Orders and Meds:

SPECIFIC THERAPY OF MENINGITIS AND ENCEPHALITIS

Streptococcus pneumoniae:
-Penicillin G 250000 U/kg/d IV q4h x 10d, max 24 MU/d (NOTE: Increasing incidence of penicillin resistance streptococcus pneumoniae.) **OR**
-Ceftriaxone (Rocephin) 100 mg/kg/day IV q12h, max 4 g/d **OR**
-Vancomycin 40-60 mg/kg/d IV q6h, max 2 g/d

Neisseria meningitides
-Penicillin G 250000 U/kg/d IV q4h x 7-10d, max 24 MU/d PO.

Meningococcal exposure prophylaxis (see H flu prophylaxis below):
-Ceftriaxone IM x 1 dose; <12y; 125 mg ≤12y; 250 mg **OR**
-Rifampin, <1 mth: 10 mg/kg/day PO q24h x 2 doses; >1 mth: 10 mg/kg/dose (max 600 mg/dose) PO q12h x 4 doses [150 mg, 300 mg caps, (may open capsule and sprinkle contents on food; may compound oral suspension or smaller capsules)].

Haemophilus influenzae
-Ceftriaxone (Rocephin) 100 mg/kg/d IV/IM q12 x 10d, max 4 g/d **OR**
-Cefotaxime (Claforan) 200 mg/kg/d (max 12 g/d) IV q6h x 10d **OR**
-Ampicillin (beta-lactamase negative) 200 mg/kg/d IV q6h x 10d, max 12 g/d.

H influenzae type B exposure prophylaxis & eradication of nasopharyngeal carriage: (household contacts who will be exposed to children <4 years old & non-pregnant, & all close day care contacts <2 years old):

-Rifampin 20 mg/kg (max 600 mg/dose) PO qd x 4 doses.

Group A or non-enterococcal Group D Streptococcus:

-Penicillin G 250,000 U/kg/d IV q4-6h, max 24 MU/d.

Listeria monocytogenes or Group B strep:

-Gentamicin or Tobramycin (normal renal function):

    <5 yr (except neonates): 7.5 mg/kg/d IV q8h.

    5-10 yr: 6.0 mg/kg/d IV q8h.

    >10 yr: 5.0 mg/kg/d IV q8h **AND**

-Ampicillin 200 mg/kg/d IV/IM q6h x 14d, max 12 g/d.

Staphylococcus aureus:

-Nafcillin or Methicillin 150-200 mg/kg/d IV q6h, max 12 g/d **OR**

-Vancomycin 40-60 mg/kg/d IV q6h, max 2 g/d (may require concomitant intrathecal therapy).

Herpes Simplex Encephalitis:

-Acyclovir (Zovirax) 25-50 mg/kg/d IV over 1h q8h x 21 days **OR**

-Vidarabine 15 mg/kg IV infusion over 12-24 hr daily x 10d.

Other Orders and Meds:

INFECTIVE ENDOCARDITIS

1. **Admit to:**
2. **Diagnosis:** Infective endocarditis
3. **Condition:**
4. **Vital signs:** Call MD if:
5. **Activity:**
6. **Diet:**
7. **IV Fluids:**
8. **Special Medications:**

Subacute Bacterial Endocarditis Empiric Therapy:

-Penicillin G 250,000 U/kg/day IV q4-6, max 24 MU/d **AND**

-Gentamicin or Tobramycin (normal renal function):

    <5 yr (except neonates): 7.5 mg/kg/d IV q8h.

    5-10 yr: 6.0 mg/kg/d IV q8h.

    >10 yr: 5.0 mg/kg/d IV q8h

Note: may use lower doses of aminoglycoside if strictly using for synergy.

Acute Bacterial Endocarditis Empiric Therapy (including IV drug abuser):

-Gentamicin or Tobramycin, see above **AND EITHER**

-Nafcillin or Oxacillin 150 mg/kg/d IV q6h, max 12 g/d **OR**

-Vancomycin 40-60 mg/kg/d IV q6h, max 2 g/d

Streptococci viridans/bovis:

-Penicillin G 150000 u/kg/d IV q4-6h, max 24 MU/d.

Staphylococcus aureus (methicillin sensitive):
-Nafcillin or Oxacillin 150 mg/kg/d IV q6h, max 12 g/d **AND**
-Gentamicin or Tobramycin, see above.

Methicillin resistant Staphylococcus aureus:
-Vancomycin 40-60 mg/kg/d IV q6h, max 2 g/d.

Staphylococcus epidermidis:
-Vancomycin 40-60 mg/kg/d IV q6h, max 2 g/d **AND**
-Gentamicin or Tobramycin, see above; may use lower doses if strictly using
   for synergy.

9. **Extras & X-rays:** CXR PA & LAT, echocardiogram, ECG. Cardiology and
   infectious disease consultation.

10. **Labs:** CBC, SMA 7, liver panel, ESR. Bacterial C&S x 3-4 over 24h (if
   septic, draw over 1h before starting antibiotic); MBC. Antibiotic levels. UA,
   urine C&S.

11. **Other Orders and Meds:**

ENDOCARDITIS PROPHYLAXIS

**Recommended Standard Prophylactic Regimen for Dental, Oral, or Upper
Respiratory Tract Procedures in Patients Who Are at Risk:**
-Amoxicillin: 50 mg/kg/dose (max dose: 3.0 g) given orally 1 hour before the
   procedure; then half the dose given 6 hours after the initial dose.

For Amoxicillin/Penicillin Allergic Patients:
-Erythromycin: 20 mg/kg/dose (max dose: 800 mg of erythromycin
   ethylsuccinate or 1.0 g of erythromycin stearate) given orally 2 hours
   before the procedure; then halt the dose given 6 hours after the initial
   dose **OR**
-Clindamycin: 10 mg/kg/dose (Max dose: 300 mg) given orally 1 hour before
   the procedure; then half the dose given 6 hours after the initial dose

Other Orders & Meds:

EMPIRIC THERAPY OF PNEUMONIA

1. **Admit to:**
2. **Diagnosis:** Pneumonia
3. **Condition:**
4. **Vital signs:** Call MD if:
5. **Activity:**
6. **Nursing:** Respiratory isolation. Pulse oximeter, I&O, postural percussion & drainage, nasotracheal suctioning prn. Apnea monitor for infants <1 year of age if suspected RSV.
7. **Diet:**
8. **IV Fluids:**
9. **Special Medications:**

-Humidified O2 by NC at 2-4 L/min or 25-100% by mask, adjust to keep sats >92% (or >95% if chronic lung disease is present)

Term Neonates <1 month (gram-positive cocci, group B streptococcus and occasionally Staph. aureus, and gram-negative enteric bacilli):

-Nafcillin 50-75 mg/kg/d IV q6-8h, max 12 g/d **OR**

-Ampicillin, <1 wk: 100 mg/kg/d IV/IM, q12h; >1 wk: 150 mg/kg/d IV/IM q8h **AND**

-Cefotaxime, <1 wk: 100 mg/kg/d IV q12h; >1 wk: 150 mg/kg/d IV q8h **OR**

-Gentamicin, <1 wk: 5 mg/kg/d IV q12h; >1 wk: 6 mg/kg/d IV q8h.

Children 1 month-5 years old (RSV, adenovirus, parainfluenza, S. pneumoniae, H. influenzae type B, Chlamydia trachomatous (<18 weeks), Staph aureus):

-Cefuroxime 75-100 mg/kg/d IV q8h **OR**

-Cefotaxime 150 mg/kg/d IV q8h **OR**

-Ampicillin (& gent) 200 mg/kg/d IV q6h **AND**

-Gentamicin or Tobramycin (normal renal function):

    <5 yr (except neonates): 7.5 mg/kg/d IV q8h **OR**

-Ceftriaxone 50-75 mg/kg/d IV/IM q12-24.

Oral Therapy: Treat IV until afebrile 72-96h

-Cefaclor (Ceclor), 40 mg/kg/d PO q8h, max 500 mg/dose [caps 250,500, elixir 125,250 mg/5 ml] **OR**

-Cefuroxime axetil, (Ceftin) <2 y: 125 mg PO bid; 2-12 yrs: 250 mg PO bid or >12 yrs: 250-500 mg PO bid, max 500 mg/dose [125,250,500 mg tabs] **OR**

-Loracarbef (Lorabid) 30 mg/kg/d PO q12h [100 mg/5 ml susp, 200 mg pavules] **OR**

-Cefpodoxime (Vantin) 10 mg/kg/d PO q12h [50 mg/5 ml, 100 mg/5 ml susp; 100 mg, 200 mg tabs] **OR**

-Cefprozil (Cefzil) 30 mg/kg/d PO q12h [susp 125 mg/5 ml, 250 mg/5 ml; tabs 250 mg, 500 mg] **OR**

-Cefixime (Suprax) 8 mg/kg/d PO qd-bid, max 400 mg/dose [tabs 200,400;

100 mg/ml (suspension results in higher levels than tabs)] **OR**

-Amoxicillin/clavulanate (Augmentin) 30-40 mg/kg/d of amoxicillin PO q8h x 7-10d, max 500 mg/dose [tabs 125,250,500, elixir 125, 250 mg/5 ml] **OR**

-TMP/SMX (Bactrim, Septra), 6-12 mg TMP/kg/d & 30-60 mg/kg/d SMX PO q12h [40 mg/200 mg/5 ml; DS tabs 160 mg TMP/800 mg SMX; SS tabs 80 mg TMP/400 mg SMX].

Community acquired pneumonia 5-18 years old (viral, M pneumoniae, chlamydia pneumoniae, pneumococcus, legionella):

-Erythromycin estolate (Ilosone) 30-50 mg/kg/d IV or PO q6h (not adults)[susp 125,250 mg/5 ml; tabs 125, 250, 500 mg] **OR**

-Cefuroxime 75-100 mg/kg IV q8h, max 9 g/d **OR**

-Doxycycline (Vibramycin) (>8 yrs) 5 mg/kg/d IV bid x 1d, then 5 mg/kg/d PO q12h [tabs or caps 50, 100 mg; syrup 50 mg/5 ml; susp 25 mg/5 ml]

Immunosuppressed, neutropenic Pneumonia (s. pneumoniae, gp A strep, H flu, gram neg enterics, klebsiella, mycoplasma pneumonia, legionella, Chlamydia pneumoniae, S aureus):

-Tobramycin (normal renal function):

    <5 yr (except neonates): 7.5 mg/kg/d IV q8h.

    5-10 yr: 6.0 mg/kg/d IV q8h.

    >10 yr: 5.0 mg/kg/d IV q8h **AND**

    Ticarcillin/clavulanate (Timentin) 200-300 mg/kg/d of ticarcillin IV q4-6h, max 18 g/d.

CYSTIC FIBROSIS EXACERBATION (P aeruginosa):

-Ticarcillin/clavulanate (Timentin) 200-300 mg/kg/d of ticarcillin IV q4-6h, max 18 g/d **OR**

-Ticarcillin 200-300 mg/kg/d IV q4-6h, max 24 g/d **AND**

-Tobramycin, see above **OR**

-Ceftazidime 150 mg/kg/d IV q8h, max 12 g/d

Bronchodilators:

-Albuterol (Proventil, Ventolin) (0.5%, 5 mg/cc sln) nebulized 0.01-0.03 cc/kg (max 1 cc) in 2 cc NS q1-6h and prn.

10. Symptomatic Medications:

-Acetaminophen (Tylenol) 10-15 mg/kg PO/PR q3-4h prn temp >101 or pain.

11. Extras & X-rays: CXR PA, LAT, PPD.

12. Labs: CBC, SMA 7, ABG. Blood C&S. Sputum gram stain, C&S, AFB. Antibiotic levels. Nasopharyngeal washings for direct fluorescent antibody (RSV, adenovirus, parainfluenza, influenza virus, chlamydia) & cultures for respiratory viruses. UA, C&S.

13. Other Orders and Meds:

SPECIFIC THERAPY OF PNEUMONIA

Pneumococcal pneumonia:
-Penicillin G 100,000-150,000 U/kg/d IV/IM q4-6h (max 24 MU/d) or Pen VK 25-50 mg/kg/d PO (NOTE: Penicillin resistant strains have been noted. C&S recommended.) **OR**
-Erythromycin 30-50 mg/kg/d PO or IV q6h

Staphylococcus aureus:
-Oxacillin or Nafcillin 150-200 mg/kg/d IV q4-6h x 3 weeks, max 12 g/d, then 1-3 weeks of PO **OR**
-Vancomycin 40-60 mg/kg/d IV q6h, max 2 g/d

Haemophilus influenzae:
-Ampicillin 100-200 mg/kg/d IV q6h (beta-lactamase negative); max 12 g/d **OR**
-Cefotaxime 100-200 mg/kg/d IV/IM q6-8h, max 12 g/d **OR**
-Cefuroxime 75-100 mg/kg/d IV q6-8h (beta-lactamase pos), max 9 g/d **OR**
-Ceftizoxime (Cefizox) or Ceftazidime (Fortaz) 100-150 mg/kg IV q8h **OR**

Pseudomonas aeruginosa:
-Gentamicin, Tobramycin or Amikacin, see above **AND**
-Piperacillin or Ticarcillin 200-300 mg/kg/d IV q4-6h, max 24 g/d **OR**
-Azlocillin 450 mg/kg/d IV q4-6h, max 24 g/d **OR**
-Mezlocillin 200-300 mg/kg/day IV divided q6h **OR**
-Ceftazidime 100-150 mg/kg IV q8h **OR**

Mycoplasma pneumoniae:
-Erythromycin 30-50 mg/kg/d PO or IV q6h x 14-21 days, max dose 2 gm/24h **OR**
-Tetracycline (**>8 yrs only**) 20-30 mg/kg/d IV q8-12h or 25-50 mg/kg/d PO q6h x 14-21 days.

Moraxella (Branhamella) catarrhalis:
-Cefuroxime 75-150 mg/kg/d IV q8h, max 9 g/d **OR**
-Erythromycin 30-50 mg/kg/d IV or PO q6h x 21 days **OR**
-Trimethoprim/SMX (Bactrim) 6-12 mg TMP/kg/d & 30-60 mg/kg/d SMX PO/IV q12h [40 mg/200 mg/5 ml; DS tabs 160 mg TMP/800 mg SMX; SS tabs 80 mg TMP/400 mg SMX].

Chlamydia pneumoniae (TWAR), psittaci, trachomatous:
-Erythromycin 30-50 mg/kg/d IV q6h.

Influenza A:
-Amantadine (Symmetrel) 1-9 yr: 4.4-8.8 mg/kg/d PO qd-bid (max 150 mg/d); >9 yrs: 100-200 mg/d PO qd-bid x 7d [syrup 50 mg/5 ml, 100 mg cap].

Other Orders and Meds:

BRONCHIOLITIS

1. **Admit to:**
2. **Diagnosis:** Bronchiolitis
3. **Condition:**
4. **Vital signs:** Call MD if:
5. **Activity:**
6. **Nursing:** Pulse oximeter, peak flow rate. Apnea monitor prn. Respiratory isolation.
7. **Diet:**
8. **IV Fluids:**
9. **Special Medications:**
   -Oxygen, humidified 1-4 L/min by NC or 40-60% by mask, keep sat >92%, or >95% if history of chronic lung disease.

Nebulized Beta 2 Agonists:
   -Albuterol (Ventolin, Proventil) (0.5%, 5 mg/cc sln) nebulized 0.01-0.03 cc/kg (max 1 cc) in 2 cc NS q1-4h & prn.

Respiratory Syncytial Virus (severe disease or underlying cardiopulmonary disease):
   -Ribavirin 6 g vial (20 mg/ml) in water, aerosolized by SPAG nebulizer over 18-20h qd x 3-5 days.

Influenza A:
   -Amantadine (Symmetrel) 1-9 yr: 4.4-8.8 mg/kg/d PO qd-bid (max 150 mg/d); >9 yrs: 100-200 mg/d PO qd-bid x 7d [syrup 50 mg/5 ml, 100 mg cap].

PERTUSSIS:
   -Erythromycin estolate 30-50 mg/kg/d IV or PO q6h x 10 days

Oral Beta 2 Agonists and Acetaminophen:
   -Albuterol liquid (Proventil, Ventolin) 0.1-0.2 mg/kg/dose (max 2 mg per dose if <12 yr) PO q6-8h [2 mg/5 ml or 2,4 mg tabs]
   -Acetaminophen (Tylenol) 10-15 mg/kg PO/PR q4-6h prn.

10. **Extras & X-rays:** CXR, sweat test.
11. **Labs:** CBC, SMA 7, CBG/ABG. Blood C&S, UA, C&S. Urine antigen screen. Nasopharyngeal washings for direct fluorescent antibody (RSV, pertussis, adenovirus, parainfluenza, influenza virus, chlamydia), viral and pertussis cultures.
12. **Other Orders and Meds:**

CROUP

1. **Admit to:**
2. **Diagnosis:** Croup
3. **Condition:**
4. **Vital signs:** Call MD if:
5. **Activity:**
6. **Nursing:** Pulse oximeter, laryngoscope & endotracheal tube at bedside. Respiratory isolation. Quiet room, accurate I&O's
7. **Diet:**
8. **IV Fluids:**
9. **Special Medications and Treatment:**
   -Etiologies: parainfluenza 1, 2, 3; respiratory syncytial virus; influenza A.
   -Oxygen, cool mist, 1-2 L/min by NC or 40-60% by mask, keep sat >92%.
   -Racemic Epinephrine (2.25% sln) 0.05 ml/kg/dose (max 0.5 cc) in 2-3 ml NS nebulized q1-6h.
   -Dexamethasone (Decadron) 0.25-0.5 mg/kg/dose IM/IV q6h prn; max dose 10 mg.
   -Acetaminophen (Tylenol) 10-15 mg/kg PO/PR q4-6h prn temp > 101 or pain.
10. **Extras & X-rays:** CXR PA & LAT, lateral & PA neck.
11. **Labs:** CBC, CBG/ABG. Blood C&S, UA, C&S. Urine antigen screen. Nasopharyngeal washings for direct fluorescent antibody (RSV, adenovirus, parainfluenza, influenza virus, chlamydia) & viral cultures.
12. **Other Orders and Meds:**

PNEUMOCYSTIS CARINII PNEUMONIA IN AIDS

1. **Admit to:**
2. **Diagnosis:**
3. **Condition:**
4. **Vital signs:** Call MD if:
5. **Activity:**
6. **Nursing:** Daily weights. Strict body fluid precautions.
7. **Diet:**
8. **IV Fluids:**
9. **Special Medications:**

PNEUMOCYSTIS CARINII PNEUMONIA:
   -Oxygen PRN FOR HYPOXIA
   -Trimethoprim/SMX, 20 mg TMP/kg/d IV q6h x 14-21 d [inj 16 mg TMP/ml, 80 SMX mg/ml] **OR**
   -Pentamidine isethionate 4 mg/kg/24h IV over 1-2h qd for 14-21d

PCP Prophylaxis (previous PCP or other AIDS-defining condition, CD4<200, all <1 yrs):

   -Trimethoprim/SMX DS 150 mg TMP/m^2 and 750 mg SMX/m^2/d divided bid for 3 consecutive days of week. [40 mg TMP/200 mg SMX/5 ml; DS 160 mg TMP/800 mg SMX; SS 80 mg TMP/400 mg SMX] **OR**

   -Pentamidine, >5 yrs: 300 mg via Respirgard II nebulizer over 20-30 min q month; may pretreat with Albuterol 0.01-0.03 cc/kg (max dose 1 cc of 0.5% soln).

HIV Antiviral Therapy:

   -Zidovudine (Retrovir, AZT) 90-180 mg/m^2/dose PO q6h (max 200 mg/dose); >12 yr-adult 100-200 mg/dose PO q4-8h [caps 100 mg, syrup 10 mg/ml].

10. **Extras & X-rays:** CXR PA & LAT, PPD with candida, mumps. MRI or CT scan to rule out toxoplasmosis.

11. **Labs:** CBC, SMA 7, ESR, LDH. Blood C&S x 2. Sputum Gram stain, C&S, AFB. Giemsa, immunofluorescence, or silver stain for pneumocystis. Serum CD4, CD8 lymphocyte count, p24 antigen, VDRL, serum cryptococcal antigen; lumbar puncture.

   Urine C&S, UA.

12. **Other Orders and Meds:**

OPPORTUNISTIC INFECTIONS IN AIDS

Candida Infections:

   -Clotrimazole troches 10 mg in mouth 5 times/24h **OR**

   -Ketoconazole (Nizoral)(oral thrush) 5-10 mg/kg/d PO bid **OR**

   -Nystatin susp. Premature infants 1 cc; infants 2 cc; children 4-5 cc. Place fluid between both buccal surfaces & give qid.

   -Fluconazole (Diflucan) 10 mg/kg IV or PO loading dose, followed by 3-6 mg/kg PO qd.

Candidiasis, invasive or disseminated disease:

   -Amphotericin B, test dose of 0.1 mg/kg (max 1 mg), followed by remainder of 1st days dose if tolerated. Initial dose: 0.25 mg/kg/d; increase by 0.25 mg/kg/d q1-2 days. Usual dose 0.5-1 mg/kg; max dose 50 mg.

   Pretreatment (except test dose) - Acetaminophen, hydrocortisone, diphenhydramine, Demerol during infusion.

Cryptococcus Neoformans Meningitis:

   -Amphotericin B 1 mg/kg/d IV qd over 2-4h x 8-12 weeks (see test dose & titration above) **WITH OR WITHOUT**

   -Flucytosine (Ancobon) 50-150 mg/kg/d PO in 4 divided doses x 4-6 weeks (maintain peak levels <120 mg/L) [250 mg, 500 mg caps; can make suspension] **OR**

   -Fluconazole (Diflucan) 3-6 mg/kg/d IV/PO qd [2 mg/ml IV; 50, 100, 200 mg tabs].

Herpes Simplex Infections:

-Acyclovir (Zovirax) (HSV) 5 mg/kg IV (10 mg/kg in visceral involvement) q8h for 7-10d.

Herpes Simplex Encephalitis:

-Acyclovir 20 mg/kg/dose PO q6h x 5 days (max 800 mg/dose) [200 mg caps, 200 mg/5 ml susp]; immunocompromised 500 mg/m^2/dose IV q8h.

Herpes Varicella Zoster

-Acyclovir 10 mg/kg IV over 60min q8h for 10 days.

Cytomegalovirus infections:

-Ganciclovir (Cytovene)(CMV), children >3 mo-adults: 5 mg/kg/dose IV over 1h q12h x 14-21d, maintenance 5 mg/kg/d IV qd or 6 mg/kg/dose IV 5 days/week (do not combine with zidovudine).

Active Pulmonary Tuberculosis:

-Isoniazid 10-20 mg/kg/d qd-bid (max 300 mg/day) x 9 months after culture negative, **AND**

-Rifampin 10-20 mg/kg/day PO qd-bid (max 600 mg/day) x 9 months after culture negative, **CONSIDER ADDING**

-Ethambutol <12 y: 10-15 mg/kg/day; >12 y: 15-25 mg/kg/day PO qd (max 2500 mg/d) PO x 2 months (if extrapulmonary disease, use pyrazinamide instead) [tabs 100,400 mg] **OR**

-Pyrazinamide 20-30 mg/kg/d qd-bid (max 2000 mg per day) PO x 2 months [500 mg tab or extemporaneous suspension].

Tuberculosis prophylaxis:

-Isoniazid 10-20 mg/kg (max 300 mg/day) PO qd x 12 months (9 months in Orange County) [syrup 10 mg/ml; tab 50, 100, 300 mg] .

Toxoplasmosis:

-Pyrimethamine (Daraprim) 2 mg/kg/d (max 100 mg/d) PO divided q12h x 3 days, then 1 mg/kg/d (max 25 mg/d) PO qd indefinitely & folinic acid 5-10 mg/d PO qd [25 mg tab], **AND**

-Sulfadiazine 100 mg/kg/d PO divided q6h x 3-4 weeks, with ample fluids [500 mg tab or extemporaneous suspension] **OR**

-Spiramycin 50-100 mg/kg/day x 3-4 weeks

Disseminated Histoplasmosis or Coccidiomycosis:

-Amphotericin B 1 mg/kg/d IV qd over 2-4h x 8-12 weeks (see test dose & titration above) **OR**

-Ketoconazole 5-10 mg/kg/d PO q12-24h, max 200 mg/dose [susp 20 mg/ml tab 200 mg].

Other Orders and Meds:

SEPTIC ARTHRITIS

1. **Admit to:**
2. **Diagnosis:** Septic arthritis
3. **Condition:**
4. **Vital signs:** Call MD if:
5. **Activity:** No weight bearing on infected joint.
6. **Nursing:** Warm compresses prn, keep joint immobilized.
7. **Diet:**
8. **IV Fluids:**
9. **Special Medications:**

Empiric Therapy for Infants 1-6 months (strep, staph, gram neg, gonococcus):

-Methicillin, Nafcillin, Oxacillin, 100 mg/kg/d IV/IM q6-8h **OR**

-Cefotaxime 100 mg/kg/d IV/IM q6h **AND**

-Gentamicin or Tobramycin (normal renal function): 30 days-6 mth: 7.5 mg/kg/d IV q8h.

Empiric Therapy for Infants 6 month-4 yr (H flu, streptococci, staphylococcus):

-Cefuroxime 75-100 mg/kg/d IV/IM q8h (preferred for H flu coverage until culture results available) **AND/OR**

-Nafcillin or Oxacillin 100-200 mg/kg/d IV q6h x ≥21d.

Empiric Therapy for Children >4 years (staph, strep):

-Nafcillin 150 mg/kg/d IV q6h x ≥21d, max 12 g/d **OR**

-Vancomycin (MRSA) 40-60 mg/kg/d IV q6h, max 2 g/d.

10. **Symptomatic Medications:**
    -Acetaminophen & codeine 0.5-1 mg codeine/kg/dose PO q4-6h prn pain [codeine 12 mg/5 ml].
11. **Extras & X-rays:** X-ray views of joint, CXR. Orthopedics and infectious disease consults.
12. **Labs:** CBC, ESR, blood C&S x 2, VDRL, PPD, UA. Antibiotic levels. Urine antigen screen (H flu).

Synovial fluid:

Tube 1 - Gram stain, C&S, fungal, AFB.

Tube 2 - Glucose, protein, pH.

Tube 3 - Cell count.

13. **Other Orders and Meds:**

PERITONITIS

1. **Admit to:**
2. **Diagnosis:** Peritonitis
3. **Condition:**
4. **Vital signs:** Call MD if:
5. **Activity:**
6. **Nursing:**
7. **Diet:**
8. **IV Fluids:**
9. **Special Medications:**

Secondary Bacterial Peritonitis (bowel perforation or appendicitis):
   -Ampicillin 100 mg/kg/d IV q6h, max 12 g/d **AND**
   -Gentamicin or Tobramycin (normal renal function):
      <5 yr (except neonates): 7.5 mg/kg/d IV q8h.
      5-10 yr: 6.0 mg/kg/d IV q8h.
      >10 yr: 5.0 mg/kg/d IV q8h **OR**
   -Ceftazidime 150 mg/kg/d IV q8h, max 12 g/d **AND**
   -Clindamycin 20-40 mg/kg/d IV/IM q6-8h **OR**
   -Metronidazole (Flagyl) 30 mg/kg/d IV q6h, max 4 g/d.

10. **Extras & X-rays:** CXR PA & LAT, abdominal ultrasound; KUB with lateral decubitus.
11. **Labs:** CBC, SMA 7, albumin, amylase, UA with micro, C&S, drug levels, liver panel; PT/PTT.

PARACENTESIS TUBE 1 - Cell count & differential (1-2 ml).
   TUBE 2 - Gram stain of sediment, C&S, AFB, fungal (3-50 ml).
   TUBE 3 - Glucose, protein, albumin, LDH, triglyceride, bilirubin, amylase, (2-5 ml red top tube).
   SYRINGE - pH, (3 ml).

12. **Other Orders and Meds:**

EMPIRIC THERAPY OF LOWER URINARY TRACT INFECTION

1. **Admit to:**
2. **Diagnosis:** UTI
3. **Condition:**
4. **Vital signs:** Call MD if:
5. **Activity:**
6. **Nursing:** I&O, daily weights; specific gravity for all voids if dehydration
7. **Diet:**
8. **IV Fluids:**
9. **Special Medications:**

Lower Urinary Tract Infection 3-6 months (E coli, S aureus):

-Treat IV x 3-5 days, then PO x 10-15 d, followed by prophylaxis: 1/3-½ dose qhs until VCUG & ultrasound done.

-Ampicillin, <1 week old: 100 mg/kg/d IV q12h **OR** >1 week old: q6-8h; max 12 g/d **AND**

-Gentamicin or Tobramycin, 7.5 mg/kg/d IV q8h **OR**

-Cefotaxime 100 mg/kg/d IV q6-8h, max 12 g/d.

Lower Urinary Tract Infection >6 months (E coli, Proteus mirabilis, S aureus):

-TMP/SMX (Septra) 6-10 mg/kg/d TMP PO q12h treat for 3,7 or 10 days [40/200/ 5 ml; DS 160/800; SS 80/400] **OR**

-Amoxicillin 30-40 mg/kg/d PO q8h x 7-10 days [tabs 125,250,500; elixir 125,250 mg/5 ml] **OR**

-Loracarbef (Lorabid) 30 mg/kg/d PO q12h [100 mg/5 ml susp, 200 mg pavules] **OR**

-Cefpodoxime (Vantin) 10 mg/kg/d PO q12h [50 mg/5 ml, 100 mg/5 ml susp; 100 mg, 200 mg tabs] **OR**

-Cefprozil (Cefzil) 30 mg/kg/d PO q12h [susp 125 mg/5 ml, 250 mg/5 ml; tabs 250 mg, 500 mg] **OR**

-Amoxicillin/clavulanate (Augmentin) 30-40 mg/kg/d of amoxicillin PO q8h x 7-10 d [tabs 250,500, elixir 125,250 mg/5 ml] **OR**

-Sulfisoxazole 120-150 mg/kg/d PO qid x 7-10d [tab 500; syrup 500 mg/5 ml] **OR**

-Nitrofurantoin (Macrodantin) 5-7 mg/kg/d PO qid [caps 25,50,100 mg; susp 25 mg/5 ml; tabs 10,100 mg] **OR**

-Cephalexin (Keflex) 50 mg/kg/d PO qid [caps 250,500; elixir 125,250 mg/5 ml] **OR**

-Cefixime (Suprax) 8 mg/kg/d PO qd [tabs 200,400; 100 mg/ml susp].

Prophylactic Therapy:

-Trimethoprim/SMX, 2 mg TMP/kg/d & 10 mg SMX/kg/d PO qhs [40/200/ 5 ml; DS 160/800; SS 80/400] **OR**

-Nitrofurantoin 1.2-2.4 mg/kg/d PO qhs [caps 25,50,100 mg; susp 25 mg/5 ml; tabs 10,100 mg] **OR**

-Sulfisoxazole 50 mg/kg/d PO qhs [tab 500; syrup 500 mg/5 ml].

10. Symptomatic Medications:

-Phenazopyridine (Pyridium), children 6-12 yrs: 12 mg/kg/d PO tid (max 200 mg/dose), for 2 days; >12 yrs: 200 mg PO tid prn dysuria [100, 200 mg tabs].

11. Extras & X-rays: Renal ultrasound. Voiding cystourethrogram 3 weeks after infection.

12. Labs: CBC, SMA 7. UA with micro, urine Gram stain, C&S. Repeat urine C&S 24-48 hours after therapy, AFB, blood C&S drug levels. ESR.

13. Other Orders and Meds:

PYELONEPHRITIS

1. Admit to:

2. Diagnosis: Pyelonephritis

3. Condition:

4. Vital signs: Call MD if:

5. Activity:

6. Nursing: I&O, daily weights

7. Diet:

8. IV Fluids:

9. Special Medications:

-If less than 1 week old, see "rule out sepsis," page 29.

-Gentamicin or Tobramycin (normal renal function):

30 days-5 yr: 7.5 mg/kg/d IV q8h.

5-10 yr: 6.0 mg/kg/d IV q8h.

>10 yr: 5.0 mg/kg/d IV q8h **AND EITHER**

-Ampicillin, >1 week: 100 mg/kg/d IV q6h, max 12 g/d **OR**

-Ticarcillin/clavulanic acid (Timentin) 200-300 mg/kg/d of ticarcillin IV q4-6h, max 18 g/d **OR**

-Trimethoprim/Sulfamethoxazole (Septra DS) 20 mg of TMP/kg/24h IV divided q6-8h (max dose 320 mg/24h); x 10d [40/200/ 5 ml; DS 160/800; SS 80/400] **OR**

-Ceftriaxone (Rocephin) 50-75 mg/kg/d IV/IM q12-24h, max 4 g/d **OR**

-Cefotaxime 100 mg/kg/d IV q8h, max 12 g/d.

10. Symptomatic Medications:

-Phenazopyridine (Pyridium), children 6-12 yrs: 12 mg/kg/d PO tid prn dysuria (max 200 mg/dose); >12 yrs: 200 mg PO tid prn dysuria [100, 200 mg].

11. Extras & X-rays: Renal ultrasound. Voiding cystourethrogram at completion of therapy.

12. Labs: CBC, SMA 7, ESR. UA with micro, urine, C&S. Repeat urine C&S 24-48 hours after therapy; blood C&S; drug levels peak & trough 3rd dose.

13. Other Orders and Meds:

OSTEOMYELITIS

1. **Admit to:**
2. **Diagnosis:** Osteomyelitis
3. **Condition:**
4. **Vital signs:** Call MD if:
5. **Activity:**
6. **Nursing:** Keep involved extremity elevated and immobilized.
7. **Diet:**
8. **IV Fluids:**
9. **Special Medications:**

Neonates, Empiric Therapy (Staph, gram neg, gp B strep):
-Methicillin 50-75 mg/kg/d IV/IM q8h **OR/AND**
-Nafcillin 100-150 mg/kg/d IV/IM q8h **AND**
-Cefotaxime 100-150 mg/kg/d IV q8h **OR**
-Ceftriaxone (Rocephin) 50-75 mg/kg/d IV/IM q12-24h **OR**
-Gentamicin or tobramycin.

Infants ≤3 yrs (H flu, strep):
-Cefuroxime 100-150 mg/kg/d IV/IM q8h **OR**
-Ceftriaxone (Rocephin) 50-75 mg/kg/d IV/IM q12-24h.

Children >3 yrs (staph, strep, H flu):
-Nafcillin 100-150 mg/kg/d IV q6h, max 12 g/d **OR**
-Cefazolin (Ancef) 100 mg/kg/d IV/IM q6-8h, max 6 g/d **OR**
-Cefuroxime 100-150 mg/kg/day IV/IM divided q8h

Postoperative or Trauma (staph, gram neg, Pseudomonas):
-Ticarcillin/Clavulanate (Timentin) 200-300 mg/kg/d of ticarcillin IV q4-6h, max 18 g/d **OR**
-Vancomycin (MRSA) 40-60 mg/kg/d IV q6h, max 2 g/d **AND**
-Ceftriaxone (Rocephin) 50-75 mg/kg/d IV/IM q12-24h, max 4 g/d.
-Ceftazidime 150 mg/kg/day IV/IM divided q8h **OR**
-Mezlocillin 200-300 mg/kg/day IV divided q6h **AND**
-Gentamicin 6 mg/kg/d IV/IM divided q8h.

10. **Symptomatic Medications:**
-Meperidine (Demerol) 1-1.5 mg/kg/dose IV/IM q3-4h prn pain.

11. **Extras & X-rays:** Technetium & Gallium bone scans, multiple X-ray views, CT/MRI. Orthopedic & infectious disease consultations.

12. **Labs:** CBC, SMA 7, blood C&S x 3, MIC, MBC, ESR, sickle prep, UA, C&S. Antibiotic levels.

13. Other Orders and Meds:

OTITIS MEDIA & EXTERNA

Acute Otitis Media (S pneumoniae, non-typable H flu, M catarrhalis, Staph a, group A strep):
- Treatment (10-14 days)
- Amoxicillin 30-40 mg/kg/d PO q8h [tabs 125,250 mg; caps 250,500 mg; susp 125,250 mg/5 ml] **OR**
- Trimethoprim/SMX 6-8 mg/kg/d of TMP PO q12h or 1 ml/kg/d PO divided bid [40/200/ 5 ml; DS 160/800; SS 80/400] **OR**
- Erythromycin/Sulfisoxazole (Pediazole) 1 ml/kg/d or 40-50 mg/kg/d of erythromycin PO q6h [erythromycin ethylsuccinate 200 mg/ sulfisoxazole 600 mg/5 ml] **OR**
- Amoxicillin/clavulanate (Augmentin) 20-40 mg/kg/d of amoxicillin PO q8h [tabs 250,500, elixir 125,250 mg/5 ml] **OR**
- Cefaclor (Ceclor) 40 mg/kg/d PO q8h [tabs 250,500; elixir 125,250 mg/5 ml] **OR**
- Cefixime (Suprax) 8 mg/kg PO qd or 4 mg/kg q12h [susp, 100 mg/ml] **OR**
- Cefuroxime axetil (Ceftin) <12 yrs: 125-250 mg PO bid; >12 yrs: 250-500 mg PO bid [125,250,500 mg tabs] **OR**
- Loracarbef (Lorabid) 30 mg/kg/d PO q12h [100 mg/5 ml susp, 200 mg pavules] **OR**
- Cefpodoxime (Vantin) 10 mg/kg/d PO q12h [50 mg/5 ml, 100 mg/5 ml susp; 100 mg, 200 mg tabs] **OR**
- Cefprozil (Cefzil) 30 mg/kg/d PO q12h [susp 125 mg/5 ml, 250 mg/5 ml; tabs 250 mg, 500 mg] **OR**
- Ampicillin 50-80 mg/kg/d PO q6h [tabs 125,250 mg caps 250,500 mg; elixir 125, 250 mg/5 ml].

Prophylactic Therapy (≥3 episodes in 6 months):
- Sulfisoxazole (Gantrisin) 50 mg/kg/d PO qhs [tab 500; susp 500 mg/500 ml] **OR**
- Amoxicillin 20 mg/kg/d PO qhs [caps 250,500 mg; suspension 125,250 mg/5 ml] **OR**
- Trimethoprim/SMX 4 mg/kg/d of TMP & 20 mg/kg/d of SMX PO qhs [40/200/ 5 ml; DS 160/800; SS 80/400].

Otitis Externa (Pseudomonas, gram neg, proteus):
- Polymyxin B/neomycin/hydrocortisone (Cortisporin otic susp) 2-4 drops in ear canal tid-qid x 5-7 days.

Malignant Otitis Externa in Diabetes (Pseudomonas):
- Ceftazidime 100-150 mg/kg/d IV q8h, max 12 g/d **OR**
- Piperacillin, Ticarcillin, or Azlocillin 200-300 mg/kg/d IV q4-6h, max 24 g/d.

Symptomatic Therapy:
- Acetaminophen 10-15 mg/kg PO/PR q4h [325, 500 mg tabs; 80 mg chewable tabs; 160 mg caplets; 80 mg/0.8 ml drops; 160 mg/5 ml elixir; 160 mg/5 ml syrup] **OR**
- Acetaminophen & codeine 0.5-1 mg codeine/kg/dose PO q4-6h prn pain [codeine 12 mg/5 ml].
- Benzocaine/antipyrine (Auralgan otic) fill canal & insert saturated pledget tid-qid prn pain x 2-3 days. Contraindicated in tympanic perforation.

Extras & X rays: sinus series, tympanocentesis, tympanogram; audiometry evaluation and testing. Unresponsive cases may require ENT consult for tympanostomy and tube placement.

Other Orders and Meds:

PHARYNGEAL INFECTIONS

1. Therapy:
STREPTOCOCCAL PHARYNGITIS
- Benzathine Penicillin (Bicillin) 25000 U/kg (max 1.2 mu) IM x 1 dose **OR**
- Penicillin V 40 mg/kg/d PO q6h x 10 days [tabs 125, 250,500; elixir 125,250 mg/5 ml] **OR**
- Erythromycin estolate (Ilosone) (penicillin allergic patients) 40 mg/kg/d PO q6h x 10 days (not adults) [elixir 125,250 mg/5 ml; tabs 125, 250; 500 mg] **OR**
- Clarithromycin (Biaxin)15 mg/kg/day PO q12h [250, 500 mg tab]

Refractory Pharyngitis (Gp A strep, viruses, N. gonorrhoea):
- Penicillin V x 10 days plus Rifampin 10 mg/kg PO q12h for last 4 days **OR**
- Amoxicillin/clavulanate (Augmentin) 30-40 mg/kg/d PO q8h [tabs 250,500; suspension 25,250 mg/5 ml] **OR**
- Dicloxacillin 50-100 mg/kg/d PO q6h [caps 125,250,500; elixir 62.5 mg/5 ml] **OR**
- Cephalexin (Keflex) 25-50 mg/kg/d PO q6-12h [caps 250, 500 mg; susp 125,250 mg/5 ml].

Prophylaxis (5 strep infection in 6 months):
- Penicillin V 25-50 mg/kg/d PO bid [tabs 125,250,500 mg; susp 125,250 mg/5 ml].

RETROPHARYNGEAL ABSCESS or Cellulitis (strep, anaerobes, E corrodens):
- Clindamycin 30-40 mg/kg/d IV/IM q6-8h, max 2.7 g/d **OR**
- Nafcillin 100-150 mg/kg/d IV q6h, max 12 g/d **OR**
- Cefuroxime 75-100 mg/kg/d IV q8h, max 9 g/d

2. Labs:
Throat culture, rapid antigen test; lateral & PA neck films; CXR. Otolaryngology consult for possible incision & drainage.

3. Other Orders and Meds:

EPIGLOTTITIS

1. **Admit to:** Pediatric intensive care unit.
2. **Diagnosis:** Epiglottitis
3. **Condition:**
4. **Vital signs:** Call MD if:
5. **Activity:**
6. **Nursing:** Pulse oximeter. Keep head of bed elevated, allow patient to sit; curved blade laryngoscope, oropharyngeal tube at bedside. Avoid excessive manipulation or agitation. Respiratory isolation.
7. **Diet:** NPO
8. **IV Fluids:**
9. **Special Medications:**
   -Note: A definitive airway should be secured before manipulation of the patient.
   -Oxygen, humidified, blow-by, keep sat >92%.
   -Cool mist humidifier tent.

Antibiotics (H flu type b, S. pneumoniae):
   -Cefuroxime 75-100 mg/kg/d IV/IM q8h, max 9 g/d **OR**
   -Ceftriaxone 50-75 mg/kg/d IV/IM q12-24h, max 4 g/d **OR**
   -Cefotaxime 100-150 mg/kg/d IV/IM q6-8h, max 12 g/d **OR**
   -Acetaminophen (Tylenol) 10-15 mg/kg PR q4-6h prn temp >38.5 or pain.
10. **Extras & X-rays:** CXR PA & LAT, lateral neck (soft tissue). Otolaryngology consult.
11. **Labs:** CBC, CBG/ABG. Blood & throat C&S, latex agglutination; UA, C&S. Urine antigen screen.
12. **Other Orders and Meds:**

SINUSITIS

1. **Treatment of Sinusitis (S. pneumoniae, H flu, M catarrhalis, gp A strep, anaerobes):**
   -Treatment 14-21 days.
   -Amoxicillin 30-40 mg/kg/d PO q8h [tabs 125,250,500; elixir 125,250 mg/5 ml] **OR**
   -Trimethoprim/SMX 6-8 mg/kg/d of TMP PO q12h [40/200/ 5 ml; DS tab 160/800; SS tab 80/400] **OR**
   -Amoxicillin/clavulanate (Augmentin) 30-40 mg/kg/d of amoxicillin PO q8h

[tabs 250,500, elixir 125,250 mg/5 ml] **OR**
- Erythromycin/Sulfisoxazole (Pediazole) 1-1.25 ml/kg/d PO q6h or 40-50 mg/kg/d of erythromycin PO q6h [erythromycin ethylsuccinate 200 mg/5 ml] **OR**
- Cefaclor (Ceclor) 40 mg/kg/d PO q8h [caps 250,500 mg; elixir 125,250 mg/5 ml] **OR**
- Cefixime (Suprax) 8 mg/kg PO qd or 4 mg/kg q12h [tabs 200,400 mg; 100 mg/ml] **OR**
- Cefuroxime axetil (Ceftin) <12 yrs: 125-250 mg PO bid; >12 yrs: 250-500 mg PO bid [tabs 125,250,500 mg] **OR**
- Ampicillin 50-80 mg/kg/d PO qid [caps 250,500 mg; elixir 125, 250 mg/5 ml].

2. **Other Meds:**
3. **Labs:** Sinus x-rays (unreliable in children <5 yrs due to incomplete development of sinuses). CBC, ESR. ENT consult for refractory cases for culture of sinus cavities.

ACTIVE PULMONARY TUBERCULOSIS

1. **Admit to:**
2. **Diagnosis:** Active Pulmonary Tuberculosis
3. **Condition:**
4. **Vital signs:**
5. **Activity:**
6. **Nursing:** Respiratory isolation.
7. **Diet:**
8. **Special Medications:**

Pulmonary Infection:

6 Month Regimen: Two months of isoniazid, rifampin, pyrazinamide daily, followed by 4 months of isoniazid and rifampin daily **OR**

Two months of isoniazid, rifampin, pyrazinamide daily followed by 4 months of isoniazid and rifampin twice weekly.

9 Month Regimen (alternative): Nine months of isoniazid, and rifampin daily **OR**

One month of isoniazid and rifampin daily, followed by 8 months of isoniazid and rifampin twice weekly.

Dosages of Anti-tuberculosis Agents:
- Isoniazid, daily dose: 10 mg/kg/d PO qd (max 300 mg).
  Twice weekly dose: 20-40 mg/kg (max 900 mg).
- Rifampin, daily dose: 10-15 mg/kg/d PO qd (max 600 mg).
  Twice weekly dose: 10-20 mg/kg PO qd (max 600 mg).
- Pyrazinamide 20-30 mg/kg PO qd (max 2000 mg).

Tuberculosis Prophylaxis for skin test conversion (Positive PPD, no disease):
- -Isoniazid-susceptible, 10-15 mg/kg/d (max 800 mg) PO qd x 9 months.
- -Isoniazid-resistant: 9 months of daily Rifampin, 10-15 mg/kg/d PO qd (max 600 mg).

9. **Extras & X-rays:** CXR PA, LAT & lordotic views, spinal series, ECG.
10. **Labs:** CBC, SMA7, liver panel, HIV (ELISA), ABG. First AM sputum for AFB x 3, Gastric aspirates qAM x 3. UA, C&S.
11. **Other Orders and Meds:**

CELLULITIS

1. **Admit to:**
2. **Diagnosis:** Cellulitis
3. **Condition:**
4. **Vital signs:** Call MD if:
5. **Activity:**
6. **Nursing:** Keep affected extremity elevated; warm compresses qid prn.
7. **Diet:**
8. **IV Fluids:**
9. **Special Medications:**

SCALDED SKIN SYNDROME, IMPETIGO, STAPHYLOCOCCAL SCARLET FEVER:
- -Oxacillin or Nafcillin 100-200 mg/kg/d IV q4-6h, max 12 g/d **OR**
- -Dicloxacillin (after response to IV Tx) 25-50 mg/kg/d PO qid x 5-7d [caps 125,250,500 mg; elixir 62.5 mg/5 ml] **OR**
- -Erythromycin estolate 40-50 mg/kg/d PO q6h [elixir 125,250 mg/5 ml; tabs 125, 250; 500 mg] **OR**
- -Cephalexin (Keflex) 25-50 mg/kg/d PO q6h [caps 250, 500 mg; elixir 125,250 mg/5 ml] **OR**
- -Loracarbef (Lorabid) 30 mg/kg/d PO q12h [100 mg/5 ml susp, 200 mg pavules] **OR**
- -Cefpodoxime (Vantin) 10 mg/kg/d PO q12h [50 mg/5 ml, 100 mg/5 ml susp; 100 mg, 200 mg tabs] **OR**
- -Cefprozil (Cefzil) 30 mg/kg/d PO q12h [susp 125 mg/5 ml, 250 mg/5 ml; tabs 250 mg, 500 mg] **OR**
- -Mupirocin (Bactroban) gel, apply topically tid. Extensive involvement requires systemic antibiotics.

Empiric Therapy Extremity Cellulitis:
- -Nafcillin or Oxacillin 100-200 mg/kg/d/IV q4-6h, max 12 g/d **OR**
- -Cefazolin (Ancef) 75-100 mg/kg/d IV/IM q6-8h, max 6 g/d **OR**
- -Cefoxitin (Mefoxin) 100-150 mg/kg/d IV/IM q6h, max 12 g/d **OR**

-Ticarcillin/clavulanate (Timentin) 200-300 mg/kg/d IV/IM q4-6h, max 18 g/d **OR**

-Dicloxacillin 50-100 mg/kg/d PO qid [caps 125,250,500; elixir 62.5 mg/5 ml].

Cheek/Buccal Cellulitis (H flu):

-Cefuroxime 75-100 mg/kg/d IV q8h, max 9 g/d **OR**

-Cefotaxime 100-150 mg/kg/d IV/IM q6-8h, max 12 g/d.

ERYSIPELAS, STREPTOCOCCAL:

-Benzathine penicillin G (Bicillin) 25,000-50,000 U/kg/dose IM x 1 dose **OR**

-Penicillin V 25-50 mg/kg/d PO q6h x 10d [tabs 125,250, 500 mg; elixir 125,250 mg/5 ml]

PERIORBITAL CELLULITIS (H. flu, pneumococcus; consider lumbar puncture, especially in unimmunized children):

-Cefuroxime 100 mg/kg/d IV/IM q8h, max 9 g/d.

10. Symptomatic Medications:

-Acetaminophen & codeine 0.5-1 mg codeine/kg/dose PO q4-6h prn pain [codeine 12 mg/5 ml].

-Codeine 0.5-1 mg/kg/dose PO/IM/SC q4-6h.

11. Extras & X-rays: X-ray views of site, Technetium/Gallium scan.

12. Labs: CBC, SMA 7, blood C&S, ESR. Leading edge aspirate, drainage fluid for Gram stain C&S; UA, urine C&S.

13. Other Orders and Meds:

TETANUS PROPHYLAXIS

History of One or Two Primary Immunizations or Unknown:

Low risk wound - Tetanus toxoid 0.5 ml IM.

Tetanus prone - Tetanus toxoid 0.5 ml IM plus Tetanus immunoglobulin (TIG) 250 U IM.

Three Primary Immunizations and 10 yrs or more since last Booster:

Low risk wound - Tetanus toxoid, 0.5 ml IM.

Tetanus prone - Tetanus toxoid, 0.5 ml IM.

Three Primary & 5-10 yrs since last Booster:

Low risk wound - None

Tetanus prone - Tetanus toxoid, 0.5 ml IM.

Three Primary & ≤5 yrs since last Booster:

Low risk wound - None

Tetanus prone - None

PELVIC INFLAMMATORY DISEASE

1. **Admit to:**
2. **Diagnosis:** Pelvic Inflammatory Disease
3. **Condition:**
4. **Vital signs:** Call MD if:
5. **Activity:**
6. **Nursing:**
7. **Diet:**
8. **IV Fluids:**
9. **Special Medications:**

Adolescent Outpatients

-Ceftriaxone (Rocephin) 250 mg IM once **and** doxycycline as below **OR**

-Cefoxitin 2 gm IM, with Probenecid 1 gm PO with doxycycline as below **AND**

-Doxycycline (Vibramycin) 100 mg PO bid x 10-14d [tabs/caps 50, 100 mg] **OR**

-Erythromycin 500 mg PO qid x 10 days [tabs 250, 500 mg] (if doxycycline is contraindicated).

Adolescent Inpatients

-Cefoxitin (Mefoxin) 2 gm IV q6h **OR**

-Cefotetan 2 gm IV q12h **AND**

-Doxycycline (Vibramycin) 100 mg IV/PO q12h (IV for 4 days & 48h after afebrile, then complete 10-14 days of Doxycycline 100 mg PO bid) [tabs 100]. Do not use in child <8 yrs.

Gonorrhea in Children less than 45 kg:

-Ceftriaxone 125 mg IM x 1 dose (uncomplicated disease only) **OR** 50-75 mg/kg/d IV/IM q24h (ophthalmia, peritonitis, bacteremia, arthritis, treat 7 days) **OR**

-Spectinomycin 40 mg/kg IM, max 2 g x 1 dose **OR**

-Amoxicillin 50 mg/kg PO once Plus probenecid 25 mg/kg PO once (max 1 gm).

10. **Symptomatic Medications:**

-Acetaminophen (Tylenol) 10-15 mg/kg/dose PO/PR q4-6h prn.

11. **Extras & X-rays:** Pelvic ultrasound.
12. **Labs:** CBC, SMA 7 & 12, ESR. GC & chlamydia culture. UA with micro; serum beta HCG or urine pregnancy test.
13. **Other Orders and Meds:**

LICE

TREATMENT:

Disinfect clothing or bedding used in last 48-hours with hot water cycle machine washing or drying, or dry clean.

For eyelash infestation, apply ophthalmic-grade petrolatum ointment bid for 8-10 days. Nit comb remove nits.

1% Lindane (Kwell, Gamma benzene) - (cream, lotion, shampoo):

Treatment of pediculosis: apply lotion or cream to the affected hairy and adjacent areas; avoid contact with eyes, or mucous membranes. After 8-12 hours, wash with soap & water. Alternatively, 1% lindane shampoo may be used for head or pubic lice. Apply 15-30 ml of shampoo and lather for 4-5 minutes. Rinse hair with water, fine tooth comb remaining nit shells. Do NOT use shampoo for eyelash treatment. First treatment with lindane is usually successful. Treatment may be repeated after one week if live lice or nits remain. Contraindicated in children <2 years of age.

0.3% Pyrethrin with Piperonyl Butoxide (A-200, Rid, R&C) - (shampoo, gel, soln):

Apply to affected hairy and adjacent areas, avoiding face. After 10 min, wash hair with soap or shampoo; fine tooth comb remaining nits. May be repeated in 7-10 days prn.

1% Permethrin (Nix) (very effective):

Shampoo, rinse, and towel dry hair. Saturate hair and scalp with permethrin (especially behind ears, nape of neck). Allow to remain on the hair for 10 min before rinsing; single treatment is sufficient. Comb out remaining nits.

SCABIES

General Considerations:

Sarcoptes Scabies:

Bathe with soap and water; scrub and remove scaling or crusted detritus; towel dry. All clothing and bed linen contaminated within past 2 days should be hot water, washed and heat dried for 20 min or dry clean.

Treatment Regimens:

10% Crotamiton (Eurax) - cream or lotion :

For scabies treatment of infants and children ≤2 years of age, pregnant/lactating women: CDC recommends 10% crotamiton rather than lindane.

Massage a thin layer of 10% cream or lotion into skin from neck to toes (including soles). Do not apply to the face, eyes, or mucous membranes. Reapply after 24 hours. Bathe 48 hours after last application. The first treatment of is usually successful; treatment may be repeated after 7-10 days if mites or new lesions.

Contraindications: Raw or weeping skin; sensitivity or allergy to crotamiton.

1% Lindane (Kwell, Gamma benzene) - available as cream, lotion:

Use 1% lindane for adults and older children; not recommended in pregnancy, infants, or excoriated skin. One treatment is usually effective. Massage a thin layer from neck to toes (including soles). In adults, 20-30 g of cream or lotion is sufficient for 1 application. Bathe after 8-12 hours. May be repeated in one week if mites or new lesions. Contraindicated in children <2 years of age.

5% Permethrin (Elimite) - cream (Very effective):

Adults and children: massage from head to soles of feet. Remove by washing after 8 to 14 hours. Treat infants on scalp, temple and forehead. One application is curative. Persistent pruritus after treatment is not an indication for retreatment.

GASTROENTEROLOGY

GASTROENTERITIS & DIARRHEA

1. **Admit to:**
2. **Diagnosis:** Acute Gastroenteritis
3. **Condition:**
4. **Vital signs:** Call MD if:
5. **Activity:**
6. **Nursing:** I&O, daily weights, urine specific gravity.
7. **Diet:** NPO, Pedialyte or soy formula (Isomil), or bland diet.
8. **IV Fluids:** see Dehydration page 73.
9. **Special Medications:**

Gastroenteritis and Diarrhea:

Rotavirus, for supportive treatment see Dehydration page 73.

Severe Gastroenteritis with Fever, gross blood and neutrophils in stool, (C jejuni, E coli, Shigella, Salmonella):

  -Trimethoprim/SMX (not effective C jejuni) 10 mg TMP/kg/d, 50 mg SMX/kg/d PO bid x 5-7d [40 mg/200 mg/5 ml; DS tabs 160 mg TMP/800 mg SMX; SS tabs 80 mg TMP/400 mg SMX].

ANTIBIOTIC ASSOCIATED & PSEUDOMEMBRANOUS COLITIS; (Clostridium difficile):

  -Vancomycin 10-40 mg/kg/d PO qid x 7 days, max 2 g/d **OR**

  -Metronidazole 15-40 mg/kg/day PO/IV q8h x 7 days, max 4 g/d.

Salmonella (treat infants & patients with septicemia):

  -Ampicillin 100-200 mg/kg/d IV q6h, max 12 g/d **OR** 50-80 mg/kg/d PO qid x 5-7d **OR**

  -Ceftriaxone 50 mg/kg/d IV qd, max 4 g/d **OR**

  -Trimethoprim/SMX 10 mg TMP/kg/d 50 mg SMX/kg/d PO bid x 5-7d [40/200/5 ml; DS 160/800; SS 80/400] **OR**

  -Amoxicillin 30-50 mg/kg/d PO tid.

Also see "Dehydration" page 73.

Symptomatic Meds if indicated for acute, noninfectious gastroenteritis and diarrhea:

  -Kaolin with pectin (Kaopectate), 3-6 yrs: 15-30 cc/dose; 6-12 yrs: 30-60 cc/dose; >12 y: 60-120 ml/dose after each loose BM or q3-4h prn **OR**

  -Loperamide (Imodium) 0.4-0.8 mg/kg/d PO q6-12h, max 4 mg/d & 7 days [1 mg/5 cc, caps 2 mg] **OR**

  -Diphenoxylate with atropine (Lomotil) (>2 yrs) 0.3-0.4 mg/kg/d (max 15 mg diphenoxylate) PO tid-qid [2.5 mg diphenoxylate/5 ml] **OR**

  -Bismuth subsalicylate (Pepto Bismol):

    3-6 yr: 5 ml PO tid-qid.

    6-9 yr: 10 ml PO tid-qid.

    9-12 yr: 15 ml PO tid-qid.

>12 yr: 30-60 ml PO tid-qid.

11. Extras & X-rays: upright abdomen

12. Labs: SMA7, CBC, ESR; stool wright stain for leukocytes, rotazyme. Stool C&S enteric pathogens; C difficile toxin & culture, ova & parasites; occult blood. Urine specific gravity, UA, blood C&S.

13. Other Orders and Meds:

SPECIFIC THERAPY OF GASTROENTERITIS

Shigella Sonnei:
-Trimethoprim/SMX, 10 mg TMP/kg/d; 50 mg SMX/kg/d PO/IV q12h x 5 d **OR**
-Ampicillin (susceptible strains) 50-80 mg/kg/d PO q6h (max 12 g/d) x 5-7 d.

Yersinia (sepsis):
-TMP/SMX 10 mg/TMP/kg/d PO q12h x 5-7d.

Campylobacter jejuni:
-Erythromycin 40 mg/kg/d PO q6h x 5-7 days [elixir 200,400 mg/5 ml; tabs 125, 250; 500 mg] **OR**
-Tetracycline (**>8 yrs only**) 20-30 mg/kg/d IV q8-12h or 25-50 mg/kg/d PO q6h x 14-21 days.

Enteropathogenic E. coli (Travelers Diarrhea):
-Trimethoprim/SMX, 10 mg TMP/kg/d, 50 mg SMX/kg/d PO/IV q12h **OR**
-Doxycycline (not for use in children <8 yrs of age): 100 mg PO qd..

Enteroinvasive E coli:
-Neomycin 50-100 mg/kg/d PO q6-8h **OR**
-Trimethoprim/SMX see above.

Giardia Lamblia:
-Quinacrine hydrochloride 6 mg/kg/d PO q8h x 5d **OR**
-Metronidazole (Flagyl) 15 mg/kg/d PO q8h x 4 days **OR**
-Furazolidone 5-10 mg/kg/d PO qid, max 100 mg/dose (available in liquid suspension only).

Entamoeba Histolytica:
Asymptomatic cyst passers :
-Iodoquinol: 40 mg/kg/day+q8h **OR** Paromomycin: 30 mg/kg/day divided q8h **OR** Diloxanide furanoate: Presently available only through CDC.

Mild to moderate intestinal symptoms with no dysentery:
Metronidazole: 35-50 mg/kg/24 h divided qd-bid x 10 days FOLLOWED BY:
Iodoquinol: 40 mg/kg/day divided q8h **OR**
Paromomycin: 30 mg/kg/day divided q8h

Dysentery or extraintestinal disease (including liver abscess):
Metronidazole: 35-50 mg/kg/24h divided qd-bid x 10 days FOLLOWED

BY:

Iodoquinol: 40 mg/kg/day divided q8h

Other Orders and Meds:

ULCERATIVE COLITIS & CROHN'S DISEASE

1. **Admit to:**
2. **Diagnosis:** Ulcerative colitis/Crohn's disease.
3. **Condition:**
4. **Vital signs:** Call MD if:
5. **Activity:**
6. **Nursing:** Daily weights, I&O.
7. **Diet:** NPO except for ice chips, no milk products.
8. **IV Fluids:**
9. **Special Medications:**

Ulcerative colitis

-Sulfasalazine (Azulfidine), children >2 yrs: initial 40-60 mg/kg/d PO q4-6h; maintenance 20-30 mg/kg/d PO q6h, max 2 gm/d **OR**

-Olsalazine sodium (Dipentum) >12 yrs: 500 mg PO with food bid [caps 250 mg].

-Hydrocortisone retention enema, 100 mg PR qhs. **OR**

-Hydrocortisone acetate 90 mg aerosol foam susp PR qd-bid, or 25 mg supp PR bid.

-Prednisone 1-2 mg/kg/d PO qAM or divided bid (max 40-60 mg/d).

Crohn's disease

-Low fat, low oxalate, high calcium diet

-Prednisone 1-2 mg/kg/d PO qAM-bid, max 40-60 mg/d **OR**

-Hydrocortisone 10 mg/kg/d IV q6h, usual max 50-100 mg/dose.

-Sulfasalazine (Azulfidine), children >2 yrs: initial 40-60 mg/kg/d PO q4-6h; maintenance 20-30 mg/kg/d PO q6h, max 2 gm/d. Not used for ileal disease.

-Metronidazole 15-30 mg/kg/d PO tid (max 750-1500 mg/d).

Other Medications:

-B12, 100 mcg IM x 5d then 100-200 mcg IM q month.

-Multivitamin PO qAM or 1 ampule IV qAM.

-Folate 1 mg PO qd.

-Zinc (deficiency) 0.3 mg/kg/24h or minimum of 3 mg zinc/24h; adults: 100-220 mg/dose tid

10. **Extras & X-rays:** Upright abdomen, Surgical, GI, dietetics consults.
11. **Labs:** CBC, platelets, SMA 7, Mg, ionized calcium; liver panel, blood C&S x 2; transferrin, pre-albumin. HLA-B27. Stool C&S for enteric pathogens, ova and parasites, C. differential toxin. Wright's stain.

12. Other Orders and Meds:

PARENTERAL NUTRITION

1. **Admit to:**
2. **Diagnosis:**
3. **Condition:**
4. **Vital signs:** Call MD if:
5. **Nursing:** Daily weights, I&O; measure head circumference & height. Finger stick glucose bid when stable.
6. **Diet:**

Peripheral Parenteral Supplementation:

   -Calculate daily fluid requirement less fluid from lipid & other sources. Then calculate protein requirements: 1 gm/kg/d. Advance daily protein by 0.5-0.6 gm/kg/d until 3 gm/kg/d; monitor BUN/creatinine. Calculate percent protein to meet parenteral protein requirements:

   -Protein requirement ÷ Fluid requirement x 100 = % amino acids. Begin with maximum tolerated dextrose concentration (Dextrose concentration >12.5% requires central line).

   -Calculate max fat emulsion intake (3 gm/kg/d), and calculate vol of 20% fat required (20 gm/100 ml = 20 %):

   (weight (kg) x 4 gm/kg/d) ÷ 20 x 100 = ml of 20% fat emulsion.

   Start 0.5-1.0 gm/kg/d lipid and increase by 0.5-1.0 gm/kg/d until 3 gm/kg/d. Deliver over 18-20 hours.

   -Draw blood 4-6h after end of infusion for triglyceride.

Central Parenteral Nutrition:

   -Calculate daily protein solution fluid requirement less fluid from lipid & other sources. Calculate total amino acid requirement of 1 gm/kg/d. Advance daily protein by 0.5-0.6 gm/kg/d until 3 gm/kg/d; monitor BUN/creatinine. Then calculate percent amino acid to be infused: amino acid requirement ÷ vol of fluid from protein solution x 100. Use 15% dextrose to provide remaining volume of solution.

   -May advance daily dextrose concentration following blood glucose to 20-25% dextrose

   -Provide 60% of energy as Dextrose; Dextrose = 3.4 K cal/gm

   -Dextrose concentration >12.5% requires central line.

   -Protein: for neonates & infants start with 0.5 gm/kg/d and increase 0.5-1.0 gm/kg/d (max 10-12% of total calories/d). For children & young adults start with 1 gm/kg/d and increase 1.0 gm/kg/d (max 3 gm/kg/d).

TPN Requirements:

	Infants-25 kg	25-45 kg	>45 kg
Calories	90-120 Kcal/kg/d	60-105	40-75
Fluid	120-180 ml/kg/d	120-150	50-75
Dextrose	4-6 mg/kg/min	7-8	7-8
Protein	2-3 gm/kg/d	1.5-2.5	0.8-2.0
Sodium	2-6 mEq/kg/d	2-6	60-150 mEq/d
Potassium	2-5 mEq/kg/d	2-5	70-150 mEq/d
Chloride	2-3 mEq/kg/d	2-3	2-3
Calcium	1-2 mEq/kg/d	1	0.2-0.3
Phosphate	0.5-1 mmol/kg/d	0.5	7-10 mm l/1000 cal
Magnesium	1-2 mEq/kg/d	1	0.35-0.45
Multi-Trace Element Formula		1 ml/d	
Insulin and Acetate, if indicated.			

Multivitamin (MVI or MVC 9+3):

<1 kg	1.5 ml/d Peds MVI
1-3 kg	3.3 ml/d Peds MVI
3 kg-11 yrs	5 ml/d Peds MVI
>11 yrs	MVC 9+3 10 ml/d

Dextrose Infusion:

Dextrose mg/kg/min = % Dextrose x rate (cc/h) x 0.167/kg wt

Normal Rate: 6-8 mg/kg/min

Lipid Solution:

-Minimum of 5% of total calories should be fat emulsion (2.7% of calories as essential fatty acids). Max of 40% of calories as fat (10% sln = 1 gm/10 ml = 1.1 Kcal/ml; 20% sln = 2 gm/10 ml = 2.0 Kcal/ml).

-Neonates begin fat emulsion with 0.5 gm/kg/d & advance 0.5-1 g/kg/d.

-For infants, children & young adults begin at 1 g/kg/d, advance as tolerated by 0.5-1 g/kg/d; max 3 g/kg/d or 40% of calories/d.

-Neonates - infuse over 20-24h; children & infants over 16-20h, max 0.15 gm/kg/h.

-Serum triglyceride 6h after infusion (maintain <200 mg/dl)

8. **Extras & X-rays**: CXR, plain film for line placement, Dietetics consult.

9. **Labs:**

Daily labs - Glucose, Na, K, Cl, HCO_3, BUN, OSM, CBC, cholesterol, triglyceride, urine glucose & specific gravity.

Twice weekly Labs - Cal, phosphate, Mg, SMA-12

Weekly Labs - Protein, albumin, prealbumin, Mg, direct & indirect bilirubin, AST, GGT, alkaline phosphatase, iron, TIBC, transferrin, retinol-binding protein, PT/PTT, zinc, copper, B12, folate, 24h urine nitrogen & creatinine.

Peds Nutrition Panel I: electrolytes, glucose calcium, PO4.

Panel II: panel I and Mg, BUN, creatinine, albumin, triglycerides, AST (SGPT).

11. **Other Orders and Meds:**

GASTROESOPHAGEAL REFLUX

1. **Treatment:**
   - Thicken feedings; give small volume feedings; keep child prone with head elevated.
   - Metoclopramide (Reglan) 0.1-0.2 mg/kg/dose qid IV/PO/IM,(max 1 mg/kg/d) (give 20-30 min prior to feedings) [inj 1 mg/ml, syrup 1 mg/ml, tab 5,10 mg] **OR**
   - Cisapride (Propulsid) 0.2-0.25 mg/kg/dose PO tid-qid [10 mg scored tab] **OR**
   - Cimetidine (Tagamet) 20-40 mg/kg/d IV/PO q6h or 20-30 min before feeding [sln 60 mg/ml; tabs 200, 300,400,800 mg] **OR**
   - Ranitidine (Zantac) 2-3 mg/kg/d IV or in TPN q8h or 4-6 mg/kg/d PO q12h [tabs 150,300 mg; liquid 15 mg/ml]
2. **Extras & X-rays:** upper GI series; gastroesophageal nuclear scintigraphy (Milk scan), ph study, endoscopy.
3. **Other Orders & Meds:**

CONSTIPATION

Step-wise Treatment:

1. Child < 2 years of Age:

Glycerine suppository OR dilation with a lubricated rectal thermometer or finger is usually d that is needed in this age group.

2. Child >2 years of Age:

(1) Glycerine or bisacodyl (Dulcolax) suppository (one only)

(2) Pediatric Fleet's enema (can be repeated once)

(3) Mineral oil, 15 ml PO. Magnesium sulfate or sodium sulfate may help in passing a hard stool and softening a forming stool.

(4) Manual disimpaction, which is unpleasant for both child and physician, may be necessary.

(5) Gastrografin or Mucomyst enemas can be useful in the impaction of cystic fibrosis, but have serious potential side effects.

3. Increase Bulk End Soften the Stool, increase free water intake and use natural dietary lubricants (e.g., prune juice, olive oil, tomatoes, and tomato juice). In addition, high-residue foods (e.g., fruits and green vegetables), and the addition of bran and whole grain products are optimal for lifelong dietary changes.

4. Stool Softeners and Laxatives:

-Docusate sodium (Colace):

<3y	10-40 mg/day PO q6-24h
3-6y	20-60 mg/day PO q6-24h
6-12y	40-150 mg/day PO q6-24h
>12y	50-400 mg/day PO q6-24h

[oral soln 10 mg/ml, 50 mg/ml; caps 50,100,250 mg]

-Mineral oil:

5-11y	5-20 ml PO qd
>12y	15-45 ml PO qd

-Magnesium Hydroxide (Milk of Magnesia) 0.5 ml/kg/dose or 40 mg/kg/dose PO prn.

-Lactulose (Cephulac) Child/adolescents: 40-90 ml/24h, divided tid-qid PO; infants: 2.5-10 ml/24h, divided tid-qid PO.

-Phosphosoda enemas (Fleet's enema) repeat time 2 per night high fiber diet.

-Hyperosmotic Soln (Colyte or GoLytely) 15-20 cc/kg/h PO until bowel is clear.

5. Diagnostic Considerations: Anorectal manometry, potassium, calcium, thyroid panel. Hirschsprung's barium biopsy.

TOXICOLOGY

POISONING

DECONTAMINATION:

Activated Charcoal: 1 gm/kg/dose (max 50 gm), diluted 1:4 as a slurry, PO (first dose should be given using product containing sorbitol as cathartic). Repeat 1/2 of initial dose q4h if indicated.

Gastric Lavage: Left side down, with head slightly lower than body; place large-bore orogastric tube & check position by injecting air & auscultating. Normal Saline lavage: 15 mL/kg boluses until clear fluid (max 200-400 ml in adults), then leave activated charcoal or other antidote prn. Save initial pass for toxicological exam; contraindicated in corrosives, hydrocarbons, sharp objects.

Cathartics:

-Magnesium Citrate 6% sln:

    <6 yrs: 2-4 ml/kg/dose

    6-12 yrs: 100-150 ml

    >12 yrs: 150-300 ml

-Magnesium sulfate 10% solution 250 mg/kg.

Ipecac (not if ingestion of acid/base, caustics, tricyclics, or if obtundent, impaired gag, <6 mth, seizing):

-Ipecac syrup (give only if <1h after ingestion); 6-12 mth: 10 ml with 15 ml/kg of clear liquid; 1-12 yrs: 15 ml followed by 240 ml liquid; >12 yrs: 30 ml with 240-480 ml liquid, may repeat x 1 after 30min if no emesis.

ANTIDOTES

CYANIDE:

-Amyl Nitrate, inhale ampule contents for 30 seconds q1min until sodium nitrate is administered. Use new amp q3min **AND**

-Sodium Nitrate, 3% inj sln, 0.33 ml/kg (max 10 ml) IV over 3-5min. Repeat ½ dose 30 min later if inadequate clinical response

Followed By:

-Sodium Thiosulfate, 1.65 ml/kg of 25% sln (max 50 ml) IV, repeat ½ dose 30min later if inadequate clinical response.

NARCOTIC OR PROPOXYPHENE OVERDOSE:

-Naloxone hydrochloride (Narcan) 0.1 mg/kg/dose, max 4 mg IV/IO/ET/IM/IO may repeat q2min.

METHANOL OR ETHYLENE GLYCOL OVERDOSE:

-Ethanol 7-10 ml/kg (10% inj sln) IV over 30min, then 0.8-1.4 ml/kg/h. Maintain Ethanol level 100-150 mg/100 mL.

CARBON MONOXIDE:

-Oxygen 100% or hyperbaric oxygen if available.

PHENOTHIAZINE REACTION (EXTRAPYRAMIDAL REACTION):
    -Diphenhydramine (Benadryl) 1-2 mg/kg IV/IM q6h x 4 doses, max 50 mg/dose; followed by 5 mg/kg/24h PO for 2-3 days q6h.

DIGOXIN OVERDOSE :
    -Digibind - Digoxin immune Fab. Dose (# of 40 mg vials) =
      post-distribution digoxin level ng/ml x body wt (kg)/100 **OR**
    -Dose (mg) = mg of digoxin ingested x 0.8 x 66.7

BENZODIAZEPINE OVERDOSE:
    -Flumazenil (Mazicon) 0.01 mg/kg IV (0.1 mg/ml in 5 ml and 10 ml vials)(benzodiazepine antagonist)

ACETAMINOPHEN OVERDOSE

1. **Admit to:**
2. **Diagnosis:** Acetaminophen overdose
3. **Condition:**
4. **Vital signs:** Call MD if
6. **Nursing:** ECG monitoring, I&O, pulse oximeter, aspiration & seizure precautions.
7. **Diet:**
8. **IV Fluids:**
9. **Special Medications:**
    -Lavage with 2 L of normal saline by nasogastric tube.
    -Activated Charcoal (if indicated) 1 gm/kg PO or NG q2-4h, remove via suction prior to acetylcysteine.
    -N-Acetylcysteine (Mucomyst, NAC)(if indicated) loading 140 mg/kg PO in juice, then 70 mg/kg PO q4h x 17 doses (20% sln diluted 1:4 in carbonated beverage) (follow acetaminophen levels).
    -N-Acetylcysteine (NAC) IV dose, 20% solution, 150 mg/kg in 200 ml D5W over 15 min. Then 50 mg/kg in 500 ml D5W over 4 hours. Then 100 mg/kg in 1000 ml D5W over next 16 hours (not USFDA approved).
    -Phytonadione 5 mg PO/IV/IM/SQ (if PT >1.5 x control).
    -Fresh frozen plasma (if PT >3 x control).
10. **Extras & X-rays:** Portable CXR. Nephrology consult for possible charcoal hemoperfusion.
11. **Labs:** CBC, SMA 7, liver panel, amylase, PT/PTT; acetaminophen level now & in 4h.
12. **Other Orders and Meds:**

THEOPHYLLINE OVERDOSE

1. **Admit to:**
2. **Diagnosis:** Theophylline overdose
3. **Condition:**
4. **Vital signs:** Call MD if:
5. **Activity:**
6. **Nursing:** ECG monitoring until level <20 mcg/ml; I&O, aspiration & seizure precautions.
7. **Diet:**
8. **IV Fluids:** Give IV fluids at rate to treat dehydration.
9. **Special Medications:**
   -Activated Charcoal liquid 1 gm/kg PO q2-4h, followed by cathartic regardless of time of ingestion.
   -Charcoal hemoperfusion (serum level >60 mcg/ml, or signs of neurotoxicity, seizure, coma). Ipecac is contraindicated because may it will induce emesis and interfere with activated charcoal.

Seizure (support oxygenation & respirations): Phenobarbital or lorazepam, see page 67.

10. **Extras & X-rays:** Portable CXR, ECG.
11. **Labs:** CBC, SMA 7, theophylline level; PT/PTT, liver panel. Monitor K, Mg, phosphorus, calcium, acid/base balance, urine drug screen.
12. **Other Orders and Meds:**

IRON OVERDOSE

General Considerations and Treatment:

Induce emesis with ipecac if recent ingestion. Charcoal is not effective.

Labs: Type and cross, CBC, electrolytes, serum iron, TIBC, abdominal x-ray, PT, PTT, liver function tests, calcium. KUB x-ray to determine if tablets are present in intestines (not all tablets are radiopaque).

Toxicity:
   -Toxicity likely >60 mg/kg elemental iron.
   -Possibly toxic 20-60 mg/kg elemental iron.

Deferoxamine Challenge Test: Give deferoxamine 50 mg/kg IM, maximum 15 mg/kg. If urine turns "vin rose" color, indicates significant iron ingestion.

MANAGEMENT:

1. If hypotensive, give IV fluids, and place in Trendelenburg's position,
2. Maintain urine output of > 2 ml/kg/h.
3. Monitor electrolytes carefully. Blood products may be needed.
4. If level > 500 mcg/dl, initiate chelation therapy. If level 300-500 mcg/dl, and iron concentration > TIBC or if signs of toxicity: Begin chelation therapy.

5. Deferoxamine (Desferal) 15 mg/kg/hr continuous infusion.
6. Consider exchange transfusion in severely symptomatic patients with serum iron >1000 mcg/dl.

NEUROLOGY & ENDOCRINOLOGY

APNEA

1. **Admit to:**
2. **Diagnosis: Apnea**
3. **Condition:**
4. **Vital signs:** Call MD if
5. **Activity:**
6. **Nursing:** For neonates: Maintain isolette at neutral thermal environment. Heart rate monitor, impedance apnea monitor, pulse oximeter. Keep bag and mask resuscitation equipment at bed side. Rocker bed or oscillating water bed prn.
7. **Diet:**
8. **IV Fluids:**
9. **Special Medications:**

Apnea of Prematurity/Central Apnea:
   - Aminophylline, loading dose 5 mg/kg, then maintenance 5 mg/kg/d IV q12h
   OR
   - Theophylline loading dose 5 mg/kg x 1 dose, then 5 mg/kg/d PO q12h. Monitor levels.
   - Caffeine citrate, loading dose 10-20 mg/kg PO, then 5-10 mg/kg/d qd-bid. Note: Not commercially available in liquid form. Monitor levels.

10. **Extras & X-rays:** Pneumogram, cranial ultrasound, echocardiogram. Upper GI (rule out reflux), pH probe. EEG (rule out seizure).
11. **Labs:** CBC, SMA 7, glucose, calcium, urine drug screen. Nasopharyngeal washings for direct florescent antibody: RSV, parainfluenza, influenza, pertussis. Theophylline level, caffeine level, UA.
12. **Other Orders and Meds:**

SEIZURE & STATUS EPILEPTICUS

1. **Admit to:** Pediatric intensive care unit.
2. **Diagnosis:** Seizure
3. **Condition:**
4. **Vital signs:** neurochecks; Call MD if:
5. **Activity:**
6. **Nursing:** Seizure & aspiration precautions, ECG & EEG monitoring, pulse oximeter.
7. **Diet:**
8. **IV Fluids:**
9. **Special Medications:**

STATUS EPILEPTICUS (tonic-clonic, simple/complex partial):

1. Maintain airway, 100% O2 by mask; obtain brief history, fingerstick glucose, suction prn.
2. Start IV NS and check fingerstick glucose. If indicated, give **glucose, 1-2 ml/kg of 50% (0.25-0.5 g/kg)** IV/IO.
3. **Lorazepam (Ativan)** 0.1 mg/kg (max 4 mg) per dose IV/PR/IM **OR**
   a) **Diazepam** 0.2-0.5 mg/kg slow IV/IO (max 10 mg). Repeat q15-20min x 3 prn (max 10 mg).
   b) **Rectal Diazepam** 0.5 mg/kg (max 10 mg) PR with a small syringe 4-5 cm within rectum (use injectable product).
4. **Phenytoin** 10-15 mg/kg in normal saline at <1 mg/kg/min, max 50 mg/min IV/IO; may repeat in 20-25min to max 25 mg/kg; max 1 gm/24 hours. Monitor BP & ECG (QT interval).
5. If seizures continue, **intubate** & give **Phenobarbital** loading dose of 10-20 mg/kg IV, then 5-6 mg/kg IV q20min, max 40 mg/kg or 300 mg.
6. If seizures are refractory to above measures, general anesthesia with EEG monitoring may be necessary.

Generalized Seizures

-Phenobarbital, loading dose 10-20 mg/kg, then 3-5 mg/kg/d PO/IV qd-bid [tabs 8,16,32,65,100 mg; elixir 4 mg/ml] **OR**

-Phenytoin PO/IV loading dose of 10-15 mg/kg, then 5-7 mg/kg/d PO/IV q12-24h [caps 30,100 mg; scored chewable tabs 50 mg; elixir 125 mg/5 ml] **OR**

-Carbamazepine (Tegretol), age 6-12 yrs: initially 10 mg/kg/d PO qd-bid, increase to maintenance 20-40 mg/kg/d PO tid-qid (max 1000 mg/24h); age <6 yrs: 5-10 mg/kg/24h PO divided bid [tabs 100 mg (chewable), 200 mg] **OR**

-Valproic acid (Depakene) 10-15 mg/kg/d PO qd-tid; increase 5-10 mg/kg/d q1week to maintenance: 30-60 mg/kg/d PO qd-tid or same dose of syrup diluted 1:1 PR [caps 250 mg; syrup 250 mg/5 ml; enteric coated tabs 125-,250,500 mg] **OR**

-Primidone (Mysoline), maintenance dose: 10-25 mg/kg/d PO tid-qid [tabs

50,250 mg; susp 250 mg/5 ml].

Partial Seizure, including Secondary Generalized

-Carbamazepine (Tegretol), see above **OR**

-Phenytoin, see above **OR**

-Phenobarbital, see above **OR**

-Primidone see above **OR**

-Valproic acid, see above.

Absence Seizures

-Ethosuximide (Zarontin) initial 20 mg/kg/d PO bid; maintenance 3-6 yr: 20-40 mg/kg/d PO qd; >6 yr: 20-30 mg/kg/d PO qd, max 1500 mg/d [caps 250 mg; syrup 250 mg/5 ml] **OR**

-Valproate, 10-15 mg/kg/d PO qd-tid maintenance 30-60 mg/kg/d PO qd-tid or same dose of syrup diluted 1:1 PR

Atypical Absence, Myoclonic, Atonic

-Valproate, see above.

-Clonazepam, 0.01-0.03 mg/kg/d PO q8h initially, max 0.1-0.2 mg/kg/d PO q8h; increase q3days by increments of 0.25-0.5 mg/d.

Specific Therapies:

Hypocalcemia:

-Calcium gluconate (10%) 30-60 mg/kg (max 1 g) slow IV/IO, preferably over 1 hour.

Hyponatremia (<120):

-Hypertonic saline 3% (513 mEq/L), give ¼ of deficit over 10min & remainder over 2h (max 1 mEq/kg/h); correct to Na 125; then correct remainder of deficit over 24-48h.

Pyridoxine Deficiency:

-Pyridoxine 50-100 mg IV/IM/IO/PO qd.

10. Extras & X-rays: MRI with & without gadolinium, EEG with hyperventilation, CXR, ECG.

11. Labs: ABG/CBG, CBC, SMA 7, calcium, phosphate, magnesium, liver panel, VDRL, anticonvulsant levels. UA, drug & toxin screen.

12. Other Orders and Meds:

DIABETIC KETOACIDOSIS

1. **Admit to:** Pediatric intensive care unit.
2. **Diagnosis:** Diabetic ketoacidosis
3. **Condition:**
4. **Vital signs:** Call MD if:
5. **Activity:**
6. **Nursing:** ECG monitoring; dextrostixs q 1-2h until glucose level is <200 mg/dl, daily weights, I&O. O2 at 2-4 L/min by NC or mask. Record labs on flow sheet. Urine specific gravity.
7. **Diet:**
8. **IV Fluids:** 10-20 ml/kg 0.9% saline over 1h, then repeat until hemodynamically stable. Then give 0.45% saline, & replace ½ calculated deficit plus insensible loss over 8h, replace remaining ½ of deficit plus insensible losses over 16-24h. Keep urine >1.5 cc/kg/h.

   Add KCL when no ECG signs of hyperkalemia (peaked T), urine adequate & serum K+ ≤ 5.8 mEq/L.

Serum K+	Infusate KCL
<3	40-60 mEq/L
3-4	30
4-5	20
5-6	10
>6	0

Rate: 0.25-1 mEq KCL/kg/hr, max 1 mEq/kg/h; 20 mEq/h max.

9. **Special Medications:**
   -Insulin Regular (Humulin) 0.1 U/kg IV bolus, then 0.05-0.1 U/kg/h (50 U in 500 ml NS) continuous drip. Adjust to decrease glucose by 80-100 mg/dl/h.
   -If glucose decreases at less than 50 mg/dl/h, increase insulin to 0.14-0.2 U/kg. If glucose decreases faster than 100 mg/dl/h, continue insulin at 0.1 U/kg/h and add D5W to IV fluids. When glucose approaches 250-300 mg/dl, add D5W to IV. Change to subcutaneous when ketones resolved, HCO3 >15, and tolerating PO food; do not discontinue drip until 2h after SC dose of insulin.
   -Potassium, give maintenance plus deficit over 24h. Hold K+ if K+ is elevated or if not urinating.
   -Phosphate, consider giving K+ as 1/2 KCL and 1/2 KPO4 for first 8h, then use all KCL.
10. **Extras & X-rays:** Portable CXR, ECG. Endocrine consultation.
11. **Labs:** Dextrostixs q1-2h x until glucose <200, then q3-6h. Glucose, electrolytes q3-4h; ketones, glycosylated hemoglobin, phosphate, CBC. Anti-islet cell antibodies, anti-insulin, antithyroglobulin, antithyroid microsomal. UA, urine C&S, urine pregnancy test.
12. **Other Orders and Meds:**

NEW ONSET DIABETES

1. **Admit to:**
2. **Diagnosis:** New onset Diabetes Mellitus
3. **Condition:**
4. **Vital signs:** Call MD if:
5. **Activity:**
6. **Nursing:** Daily weights, I&O. Record labs on flow sheet. fingerstick glucose at 0700, 1200, 1700, 2100, 0200; diabetic and dietetic teaching.
7. **Diet:** American Diabetes Association Diet: with appropriate calories. 3 meals & 3 snacks between each meal & qhs.
8. **IV Fluids:** Hep-lock with flush q shift.
9. **Special Medications:**
   -Goal is fasting glucose of 70-140 mg/dl and postprandial glucose <180 mg/d
   -Initial insulin dose for child with severe hyperglycemia and ketonuria but without acidosis or dehydration: - 0.1-0.25 U regular/kg SC q6-8h.
   -On subsequent days give 2/3 of previous days total insulin requirement as NPH. Divide 2/3 before breakfast & 1/3 before dinner. Supplement with regular insulin 0.1 U/kg before each meal if indicated.
   -Usual daily maintenance dose for child: 0.5-1.0 U/kg/24h. In adolescents during growth spurt: 0.8-1.2 U/kg/24h.
10. **Extras & X-rays:** CXR. Consider endocrine consultation.
11. **Labs:** CBC, ketones; SMA 7 & 12, antithyroglobulin, antithyroid microsomal, anti-insulin, anti-islet cell antibodies; phosphate. UA, urine C&S; urine pregnancy test; urine ketones.
12. **Other Orders and Meds:**

HEMATOLOGY, NEPHROLOGY & INFLAMMATORY DISORDERS

SICKLE CELL CRISIS

1. **Admit to:**
2. **Diagnosis:**
3. **Condition:**
4. **Vital signs:** Call MD if
5. **Activity:**
6. **Nursing:**
7. **Diet:**
8. **IV Fluids:** D5½NS at 1.5-2.0 x maintenance or 2000 ml/m^2/24h.
9. **Special Medications:**
   -Oxygen 2-4 L/min by NC or 30-100% by mask.
   -Meperidine (Demerol) 1-2 mg/kg/dose max 100 mg/dose IM/IV/SC q3-4h.
   -Morphine sulfate 0.1-0.2 mg/kg/dose (max 10-15 mg) IV/IM/SC q2-4h prn
     or follow bolus by infusion of 0.05-0.1 mg/kg/h or 0.3-0.5 mg/kg PO q4h
     OR
   -Acetaminophen/codeine 0.5-1 mg/kg/dose (max 60 mg/dose) of codeine
     IM/SC/PO q4-6h prn [12 mg codeine/5 ml].
   -Cefuroxime 75-100 mg/kg/d IV q8h, max 9 g/d (or other antibiotic in
     presence of unexplained fever, toxicity, lethargy) **OR**
   -Cefotaxime 100-150 mg/kg/d IV/IM divided q8h.
   -Folic acid 1 mg PO qd (if >1 yr).
   -Transfusion (if indicated) PRBC 5 cc/kg over 2h, then 10 cc/kg over 2h, then
     check hemoglobin. If hemoglobin <6-8 gms, give additional 10 cc/kg.
   -Penicillin V (prophylaxis), <5 yrs: 125 mg PO bid, **OR** >5 yrs: 250 mg PO bid
     [tabs 125,250,500 mg; elixir 125,250 mg/5 ml]. Amoxicillin may also be
     used. Erythromycin is used in penicillin allergic patients.
   -Pneumococcal vaccination (≥2 years old), Haemophilus B, influenza
     vaccination, hepatitis B vaccination.
10. **Extras & X-rays:** CXR.
11. **Labs:** CBC, blood C&S, reticulocyte count, type & hold, hemoglobin electro-
    phoresis (if diagnosis not confirmed), parvovirus titers, SMA 7, UA, urine
    C&S.
12. **Other Orders and Meds:**

KAWASAKI'S SYNDROME
(Mucocutaneous Lymph Node Syndrome)

1. **Admit to:**
2. **Diagnosis:**
3. **Condition:**
4. **Vital signs:** Call MD if:
5. **Activity:**
6. **Nursing:**
7. **Diet:**
8. **Special Medications:**
   - Immunoglobulin (IVIG) 2 gm/kg/dose IV x 1 dose only. Administer dose at 0.02 ml/kg/min over 30 min; if no adverse reaction, increase to 0.04 ml/kg/min over 30 min; if no adverse reaction, increase to 0.08 ml/kg/min for remainder of infusion.
   - Aspirin 100 mg/kg/day PO q6h until fever resolves, then 8-10 mg/kg/day PO qd.
9. **Extras & X-rays:** ECG, echocardiogram, chest X-ray; consider angiogram prn. Infectious disease consult may be indicated.
10. **Labs:** CBC with differential and platelet count. ESR, C-reactive protein, CBC, liver function tests, rheumatoid factor, aspirin levels. Blood C&S x 2, SMA 7.
11. **Other Orders and Meds:**

FLUIDS & ELECTROLYTES

DEHYDRATION

1. **Admit to:**
2. **Diagnosis:** Dehydration
3. **Condition:**
4. **Vital signs:** Call MD if:
5. **Activity:**
6. **Nursing:** I&O, daily weights. Urine specific gravity q void.
7. **Diet:**
8. **IV Fluids:**

Maintenance Fluids:

<10 kg	100 ml/kg/24h
10-20 kg	1000 ml plus 50 ml/kg/24h for each kg >10 kg
>20 kg	1400-1500 ml plus 20 ml/kg/24h for each kg >20 kg.

If fever, increase by 10 ml/degree C/d.

Alternate Method: Calculate the sum as follows:

$$4 \text{ cc/kg (kg 1-10)} =$$
$$2 \text{ cc/kg (kg 11-20)} =$$
$$1 \text{ cc/kg (thereafter)} =$$
$$\text{(e.g.: 12 kg child = 44 cc/kg)}$$

Electrolyte Requirements:

Sodium 3-5 mEq/100 ml water required
Potassium 2-3 mEq/100 ml water required
Chloride 3 mEq/100 ml water required
Glucose 5-10 gm/100 ml water required

Clinical Fluid Deficit Status:

Mild 5-7%: Increased pulse (10% >baseline), normal blood pressure, slightly dry mucous membranes; increased thirst, decreased tears, fontanelle flat, skin turgor & eyes normal; decreased urine, increased urine specific gravity. Fluid deficit <50 ml/kg.

Moderate: Increased severity of above decreased skin turgor,
5-10% oliguria, irritability, dry mucous membranes, increased thirst, postural hypotension, elevated pulse, sunken fontanelle, absent tears, sunken eyes, increased BUN. Fluid deficit 50-100 ml/kg.

Severe: Hypotension, tachycardia, parched mucous membranes,
>10% very sunken eyes, delayed capillary refill (>3 sec), acidosis, decreased HCO3, hyperirritability, lethargy, skin tenting, anuria. Fluid deficit ≥100 ml/kg.

Electrolyte Deficit Calculation:

Na+ deficit=(desired Na-measured Na mEq/L) x 0.6 x weight Kg

K+ deficit=(desired K-measured K mEq/L) x 0.25 x weight Kg

Cl+ deficit=(desired Cl-measured Cl mEq/L)x 0.45 x weight Kg

Free H2O Deficit in Hypernatremic Dehydration = 4 cc/kg for every mEq that
serum Na> 145 mEq/L.

Phase 1 Acute Resuscitation, (Symptomatic Dehydration):

-Give D5NS or NS at 20-40 ml/kg IV over 60min; may repeat fluid boluses of
NS 10-20 cc/kg until adequate circulation (**no dextrose** in repeat boluses
unless glucose <60). If shock, give at max rate until stable.

Phase 2 Deficit & Maintenance Therapy (Asymptomatic dehydration):

HYPOtonic Dehydration (Na+ <125 mEq/L):

-Calculate total maintenance & deficit fluids & sodium deficit for 24h (minus
fluids & electrolytes given in Phase 1). If isotonic or hyponatremic
dehydration, replace 50% over 8h, 50% over next 16h.

-If hypernatremic dehydration, replace over 48h; avoid decreasing serum
sodium at a rate greater than 15 mEq/L over 24h.

-Estimate and replace ongoing losses q6-8h.

-Add potassium to IV solution after void.

-Usually D5 0.45% or 0.9% saline with 10-40 mEq/l KCL at 60 ml/kg over 2
hours. Then infuse at 6-8 ml/kg/h for 12h.

-See "hyponatremia," page 77.

ISOtonic Dehydration (Na+ 130-150 mEq/L):

-Calculate total maintenance & replacement & electrolytes fluids for 24h
(minus fluids & electrolytes given in Phase 1) and give half over first 8h,
then remaining half over next 16 hours.

-Add potassium to IV solution after void.

-Estimate and replace ongoing losses.

-Usually D5½NS or D5¼NS with 10-40 mEq KCL/L.

HYPERtonic Dehydration (Na+ >150 mEq/L):

-Calculate and correct free water deficit & correct **slowly.** Lower sodium by
10 mEq/L/d; avoid dropping Na+ by >15 mEq/L/24h or by >0.5 mEq/L/hr.

-If volume depleted, give NS 20-40 ml/kg IV until adequate circulation, then
give ½-¼ NS in 2.5-5% glucose IV to replace half of free water deficit over
first 24h. Follow **serial serum sodium levels** & correct deficit over 48-72h.

-**Free water deficit:** 4 cc/kg x (Serum Na+ -145)

-**Also see "hypernatremia" page 76.**

-If indicated, add potassium to IV solution after void as KCL or K acetate.

-Usually D5¼NS or D5W with 10-40 mEq/L KCL. Estimate & replace
ongoing losses & maintenance.

Replacement of ongoing losses (usual fluids):

-Nasogastric suction: D5½NS with 20 mEq KCL/L.

-Diarrhea: D5¼NS with 40 mEq KCL/L

Oral Rehydration Therapy (mild-moderate dehydration < 10%):

    -Oral rehydration electrolyte solution (Rehydralyte, Pedialyte, Ricelyte) deficit replacement of 60-80 ml/kg PO or via NG tube over 2h. Provide additional fluid requirement over remaining 18-20h; add anticipated fluid losses from stools of 10 cc/kg for each diarrheal stool. Avoid hypotonic solutions.

9. Extras & X-rays: CXR

10. Labs: SMA7, BUN, creatinine, glucose, urine electrolytes, UA.

11. Other Orders and Meds:

HYPERKALEMIA

1. Admit to: Pediatric ICU

2. Diagnosis: Hyperkalemia

3. Condition:

4. Vital signs: Call MD if:

5. Activity:

6. Nursing: ECG monitoring, I&O, daily weights.

7. Diet:

8. IV Fluids:

HYPERkalemia (K + >7 or EKG Changes)

    -Calcium gluconate 10% sln 0.5 cc/kg (max 10 cc) IV over 3 min; second dose may be given in 5 min. If digoxin toxicity suspected, give over 30 min or omit.

    -Bicarbonate 1-2 mEq/kg IV over 3-5 min (give after calcium in separate IV), repeat in 10-15 min if necessary.

    -Glucose 0.5 gm/kg/h **plus** insulin 1 unit regular for each 3 gm of glucose.

    -Kayexalate resin 0.5-1 gm/kg PO. 1 gm resin binds approximately 1 mEq K+
    OR

    -Kayexalate retention enema 0.5-1 gm/kg PR.

    -Consider hemodialysis.

9. Extras & X-rays: ECG, dietetics, nephrology consults.

10. Labs: SMA7, Mg, Cal, CBC, platelets. UA; 24h urine K, Na, creatinine.

11. Other Orders and Meds:

HYPOKALEMIA

1. **Admit to:** Pediatric ICU
2. **Diagnosis:** Hypokalemia
3. **Condition:**
4. **Vital signs:** Call MD if:
5. **Activity:**
6. **Nursing:** ECG monitoring, I&O, daily weights.
7. **Diet:**
8. **IV Fluids:**

HYPOkalemia

If serum K >2.5 & ECG changes are absent:

Add 20-40 mEq KCL/L to maintenance fluids. May give 1-4 mEq/kg/d as needed to maintain normal serum K+. May supplement with oral potassium.

K <2 & ECG abnormalities:

Give KCL 1-2 mEq/kg IV; recommended rate: 0.5 mEq/kg/h; max rate 1 mEq/kg/h in life-threatening situations; max 20 mEq/h. Recheck serum potassium, & repeat IV boluses prn; ECG monitoring required.

Oral Potassium Therapy (40 mEq K = 3 gm KCL):

-KCL elixir 1-3 mEq/kg/d PO [10% sln = 6.7 mEq K+/5 ml].

9. **Extras & X-rays:** ECG, dietetics, nephrology consults.
10. **Labs:** SMA7, Mg, Cal, CBC. UA, 24h urine K, Na, creatinine.
11. **Other Orders and Meds:**

HYPERNATREMIA

1. **Admit to:**
2. **Diagnosis:** Hypernatremia
3. **Condition:**
4. **Vital signs:** Call MD if:
5. **Activity:**
6. **Nursing:** I&O, daily weights.
7. **Diet:**
8. **IV Fluids:**

HYPERnatremia:

If volume depleted or shock, give NS 20-40 ml/kg IV until adequate circulation, then give D5½NS or D5¼NS IV to replace half of body water deficit over first 24h. Correct Na slowly at 0.5-1 mEq/L/h; < 12 mmol/L/d, then remaining deficit over next 48-72h.

Body water deficit (L) = $\dfrac{0.6(\text{weight kg})([\text{Na serum}]-140)}{140}$

HYPERnatremia with ECF Volume Excess:

-Furosemide 1 mg/kg IV.

-D5W or other hypotonic fluid to correct body water deficit (see above).

9. Extras & X-rays: ECG.

10. Labs: SMA 7, osmolality, triglycerides, cholesterol, albumin. UA, urine specific gravity; 24h urine Na, K, creatinine.

11.   Other Orders and Meds:

HYPONATREMIA

1. Admit to:

2. Diagnosis: Hyponatremia

3. Condition:

4. Vital signs: Call MD if:

5. Activity:

6. Nursing: I&O, daily weights.

7. Diet:

8. IV Fluids:

HYPOnatremia with increased ECF & edema (Hypervolemia)(low osmolality <280, UNa <10 mmol/L: nephrosis, CHF, cirrhosis; UNa >20: acute/chronic renal failure):

-Water restrict 1/3 - 1/2 maintenance. No added salt diet.

-Furosemide 1 mg/kg/dose IV over 1-2min or 2-3 mg/kg/d PO.

HYPOnatremia with Isovolemia (low osmolality <280, UNa <10 mmol: water intoxication; UNa >20: SIADH, hypothyroidism, renal failure, Addison's disease, Stress, Drugs):

-0.9% saline with 20-40 mEq KCL/L infused to correct at rate of <0.5 mEq/L/h) **OR** use 3% NS in severe hyponatremia.

-Water restrict to 1/3 - 1/2 maintenance.

HYPOnatremia with Hypovolemia (low osmolality <280) UNa <10 mmol/L: vomiting, diarrhea, 3rd space/respiratory/skin loss; UNa >20 mmol/L: diuretics, renal injury, RTA, adrenal insufficiency, partial obstruction, salt wasting:

-If volume depleted, give NS 20-40 ml/kg IV until adequate circulation.

-Gradually correct of Na+ deficit in increments of 10 mEq/L. Determine volume deficit clinically, & determine Na+ deficit as below.

-Calculate 24 hour fluid and Na+ requirement & give half over first 8h, then remainder over 16 hours. 0.9% saline = 125 mEq/L

-Add potassium to IV solution after void if indicated.

-Usually D5NS 60 ml/kg IV over 2h (this will increase extracellular Na by 10 mEq/L), then infuse at 6-8 ml/kg x 12h.

Severe Symptomatic HYPOnatremia:

-If volume depleted, give NS 20-40 ml/kg until adequate circulation.

-Determine vol of 3% hypertonic saline (513 mEq/L) or 5% (855 mEq/L) to be infused:

$$Na(mEq) \text{ deficit} = 0.6 \times (wt \text{ kg}) \times (\text{desired Na} - \text{actual Na})$$

$$\frac{\text{Volume of sln (L)}}{\text{(mEq/L in sln)}} = \text{Sodium to be infused (mEq)}$$

-Correct half of sodium deficit slowly over 24h.

-For acute correction, use Na 125 mEq/L as desired sodium solution; max rate for acute replacement 1 mEq/kg/hr. Serum Na should be adjusted in increments of 5 mEq/L to reach 125 mEq/L. First dose usually given over 4 hrs. For further correction for serum Na >125 mEq/L calculate mEq dose of sodium, and administer over 24-48h. Changes in Na >10 mEq/L/day not recommended

9. **Extras & X-rays:** CXR, ECG.

10. **Labs:** SMA 7, osm, trig, cholesterol, albumin. UA with micro, urine specific gravity. Urine osm, Na, K; 24h urine Na, K, Cr.

11. **Other Orders and Meds:**

HYPOPHOSPHATEMIA

Indications for Intermittent IV Administration:

1. Serum phosphate <1.0 mg/dl or
2. Serum phosphate <2.0 mg/dl & patient symptomatic or
3. Serum phosphate <2.5 & patient on ventilator

Dosage		**Serum Phosphate**
Low dose	0.08 mm/kg IV over 6 hrs	uncomplicated
Intermediate dose	0.16 IV over 6 hrs	
	0.24 IV over 4 hrs	0.5-1 mg/dl
High Dose	0.36 IV over 6 hrs	<0.5 mg/dl

Choose Cation:

NaPO4: contains sodium 4 mEq/ml, phosphate 3 mmol/ml
K phosphate: contains potassium 4.4 mEq/ml, phosphate 3 mmol/ml
Max rate 0.06 mm/kg/hr

HYPOMAGNESEMIA

IV maintenance dose MgSO4   1-2 mEq/kg/day (= 125-250 mg/kg/day)

Indications for Intermittent IV Administration:
1. Serum magnesium <1.2 mg/dl;
2. Serum magnesium <1.6 mg/dl, and patient symptomatic;
3. Calcium resistant tetany

Dosage of Magnesium Sulfate:
25-50 mg/kg/dose (0.2-0.4 mEq/kg/dose) IV every 4-6 hrs x 3-4 doses as needed (max 2000 mg = 16 mEq/dose); max rate 1 mEq/kg/hr (125 mg/kg/hr).

NEWBORN CARE

NEONATAL RESUSCITATION

APGAR (1 & 5 minutes):
Appearance: Color (0-2)
Pulse: Heart rate (0-2)
Grimace; Reflex irritability (0-2)
Activity: Muscle tone (0-2)
Respiration: Respiratory effort (0-2)
Continue assessment until APGAR ≥ 7.

General Measures:
1. Review history, check equipment, oxygen, masks, laryngoscope, ET tubes, medications.

Vigorous, Crying Infant:
1. Routine delivery room care; heart rate > 100, spontaneous respirations, good color & tone.
2. Aspirate mouth, then nose gently by bulb syringe; dry skin & maintain neutral thermal environment.

Moderate Depression:
1. If Respiratory efforts are present but skin is pale or cyanotic skin is present, provide 100% oxygen by mask or blowby.

   If **Meconium** is 2+ or more, or if respiratory distress, intubate immediately and suction trachea until clear (do not positive pressure ventilate until trachea has been suctioned).
2. If no improvement or deterioration, bag & mask ventilate with intermittent positive pressure, 100% FI02; stimulate vigorously by drying. Initial breath pressure: 30-40 cm H2O for term infants, 20-30 cm H2O pre-term. Then ventilate at 15-20 cm H20 at 30-40/min. Monitor bilateral breaths sounds and expansion.
3. If spontaneous respirations develop, normal heart rate and pulse: gradually reduce ventilation rate until only continuous positive airway pressure (CPAP). Wean to blowby oxygen, but continue blowby oxygen if baby remains dusky. Consider intubation if heart rate remains <100 beats per minute, and is not rising, or if poor or weak respiration, or for airway control.

Severe Depression:
1. Bag & mask ventilate with intermittent positive pressure, 100% FIO2.
2. If heart rate does not increase to >80/min after 30 seconds of ventilation, initiate external cardiac massage at 120 beats per min. May discontinue cardiac massage when heart rate is >80 & rising. If condition improves, change to CPAP by mask, 100% FI02, increasing to blowby oxygen.
3. If condition worsens or no change after 30 seconds, or if mask ventilation is difficult: use laryngoscope to suction oropharynx and trachea, and intubate. Apply positive pressure ventilation. Check bilateral breath sounds & chest

expansion. Check and adjust ET tube position if necessary. Continue cardiac massage if heart rate remains depressed. Check CXR for tube placement.

Hypotension or Bradycardia:

1. Epinephrine 0.1-0.3 ml/kg = 0.01-0.03 mg/kg (1:10,000) via endotracheal tube or 0.1-0.3 ml/kg (0.01-0.03 mg/kg; 1:10,000) in 1-2 cc NS IV via umbilical catheter q3-5min.
2. Atropine 0.1-0.2 ml/kg (0.01-0.02 mg/kg; 1:10,000) IV.

Hypovolemia:

1. Insert umbilical vein catheter & give O negative blood, plasma, 5% albumin, normal saline, 10 ml/kg IV. May repeat as necessary to correct hypovolemia.

Severe Birth Asphyxia, Mixed Respiratory/Metabolic Acidosis (not responding to ventilatory support; pH <7.2):

1. Sodium Bicarbonate, 1 mEq/kg, dilute 1:1 in sterile water IV q5-10min as indicated. Bicarbonate may be given for documented as well as suspected acidosis.

Narcotic-Related Depression:

1. Naloxone (Narcan) 0.1 mg/kg = 0.25 ml/kg (0.4 mg/ml concentration) IV/IM/SC/intratracheal, may repeat q15-20min. Caution: If maternal drug abuser, may cause withdrawal & seizures.

Intubation:

Premature infant <1.25 kg (2 lbs) 2.5 mm tube; size 0 blade; 7.5 cm tip to lip.
Premature 1.25-2 kg (2-5 lbs) 3 mm tube; 0 blade; 8 cm tip to lip.
Full term > 2 kg (5 lb) 3.5 mm tube; 1 blade; 8.5 cm tip to lip.

MECONIUM ASPIRATION

1. After delivery of head, clear infant nose and oropharynx with DeLee trap. Repeat DeLee suction after chest delivered.
2. Suction trachea with maximum diameter endotracheal tube with laryngoscope. If improvement, extubate & ventilate with mask or hood 100% oxygen at 40 breaths/min.
3. Suction trachea in infants with thin meconium if APGAR < 6 or if respiratory distress continues.
4. If necessary, continue mechanical ventilation and neonatal intensive care unit support.

NEONATAL SUSPECTED SEPSIS

Term Newborn Infants <1 month old (GpB strep, E coli, or GpD strep, gram negatives, Listeria monocytogenes:

Amp + cefotaxime or Amp + gentamicin;
<u>Add</u> vancomycin if >7 days old and has central line.

Neonatal Dosage of Ampicillin:
Meningitic Dose:
Age < 7 days: 200 mg/kg/d q 12h
Age >7 days: 200 mg/kg/d q 6-8h
Rule Out Sepsis Dose:
Age 7 days and weight <2 kg: 50-100 mg/kg/d divided q12h
Age 7 days and weight >2 kg: 75-100 mg/kg/d divided q12h
Age >7 days and weight <2 kg: 75-150 mg/kg/d divided q8h
Age >7 days and weight >2 kg: 100-200 mg/kg/d divided q6h

Cefotaxime:
Neonate: <1200 grams: 0-4 wks: 100 mg/kg/d divided q12h IV/IM
Neonate: > 1200 grams: 0-7 days: 100 mg/kg/d divided q12h IV/IM
>7 days: 150 mg/kg/d divided q8hr IV/IM

Gentamicin/Tobramycin: 2.5 mg/kg/dose
Dosing Interval:
Gestational Age <28 wks & < 7 days old: q24h; >7 days: q18h
28-34 wks & <7 days old: q18h; >7 days: q12h
>34 wks & < 7 days old: q12 h; >7 days: q8h

Neonatal Vancomycin Dosage Guidelines:

Wt< 1.5 kg & age <7 days:	15 mg/k/d q24h
Wt< 1.5 kg & age 7-30 days:	20 mg/k/d q12h
Wt< 1.5 kg & age <30 days:	3.0 mg/kg/d q8h
Wt 1.5-2 kg & age <7 days:	20 mg/k/d q12h
Wt 1.5-2 kg & age 7-30 days:	20 mg/k/d q12h
Wt >2 kg & age <7 days:	20 mg/k/d ql 2h
Wt >2 kg & age 7-30 days:	30 mg/kg/d q8h
Wt >2 kg & age <30 days:	40 mg/k/d q6h

Note: Vancomycin has been associated with a histaminic reaction known as "red man syndrome". If serum creatinine is >1.2 mg/dl, use an initial dosage of 15 mg/kg/day q24h and determine serum vancomycin concentrations within 24-48 hours. Post-conceptional age = gestational age & chronological age.

Nafcillin, Methicillin:
>   NEONATAL: IM, IV
>   Wt < 2 kg & Age 0-7 days: 50 mg/kg/d q 12h
>   Wt <2 kg&age> 7 days: 75 mg/k/d q8h
>   Wt >2 kg&age 0-7 days: 50 mg/k/d q8h
>   Wt > 2 kg & age • 7 days: 75 mg/kg/d q 6h

Mezlocillin:
>   <7 days: 75 mg/k/dose q12h
>   >7 days: < 2 kg: 75 mg/kg/dose q8h
>   >7 days: >2 kg: 75 mg/k/dose q6h

Amikacin: 7.5 mg/k/dose IV/IM
>   **Dosing interval:**
>   Gestational Age <28 wks and <7 days old: q24h; >7 days: q18h
>   28-34 wks <28 wks and <7 days old: q18h; >7 days: q 12h
>   >34 wks <28 wks and <7 days old: q12h; >7 days: q 8h

Laboratory Studies: CBC, SMA 7, Blood C&S; UA, C&S, antibiotic levels. CXR. Nasopharyngeal washings for direct fluorescent antibody & viral cultures. Urine antigen screen.

CSF Tube 1 - Gram stain, bacterial C&S, antigen screen (1-2 ml).

CSF Tube 2 - Glucose protein (1-2 ml).

CSF Tube 3 - Cell count & differential (1-2 ml).

RESPIRATORY DISTRESS SYNDROME

1. Provide mechanical ventilation as indicated.
2. **Exogenous surfactant:**
   - Beractant (Survanta) 4 ml/kg (birth weight) via endotracheal tube as soon as possible after clinical diagnosis made/suspected, then q6h up to 4 doses.
   - Exosurf 5 ml/kg (birth weight) (same route as above) q12h x 2-3 doses. Use birth weight for all doses

NECROTIZING ENTEROCOLITIS

Treatment:
1. Decompress bowel with a large-bore (10 or 12 French) double lumen nasogastric or orogastric tube, and apply intermittent suction.
2. Replace fluid losses with IV fluids; monitor urine output, tissue perfusion and blood pressure; consider central line monitoring.
3. Give blood and blood products for anemia, thrombocytopenia, coagulopathy.
4. Monitor abdominal X-rays for free air from perforation.
5. **Antibiotics: (Premature Infant)(E coli, Staph epidermidis, P aeruginosa, C perfringens):**
   -Ampicillin, >7 days: 100-200 mg/kg/d IV q8-12h. **AND**
   -Gentamicin or tobramycin 7-30 days old: 5-6 mg/kg/d IV/IM q8h (very premature infants require modified dosing) **OR**
   -Cefotaxime, neonate: <1200 grams: 0-4 wks: 100 mg/kg/d divided q12h IV/IM > 1200 grams: 0-7 days: 100 mg/kg/d divided q12h IV/IM >7 days: 150 mg/kg/d divided q8h IV/IM **OR**
   -Vancomycin, see dose on page 82.
6. **Diagnostic Considerations:** Serial abdominal X-ray series every 4-6 hours (with lateral decubitus), CBC with differential and platelets; DIC panel, blood cultures x 2; consider abdominal paracentesis; Wright's stain of stool; stool cultures.
7. **Frequent Evaluations:** for perforation, electrolyte disturbances, and pneumatosis intestinalis and portal vein gas (X-ray). Surgical evaluation if perforation suspected.

CONGENITAL SYPHILIS

-Penicillin G aqueous, 50,000 U/kg/dose; <1 wk - q12h; >7 d - q8h. Treat for 10-14 days. If one or more days is missed, restart entire course.

PATENT DUCTUS ARTERIOSUS

Treatment:
1. Consider fluid restriction if symptomatic, and individualize fluid therapy based on individual patient.
2. Provide respiratory support, maintain hematocrit at 40%, consider diuretics.

3. Furosemide (Lasix) 1-2 mg/kg/dose q6-8h PO **OR** 1 mg/kg/dose q12h IV is needed.

4. **Indomethacin (Indocin):**

	(mg/kg/dose)		
Age at First Dose	**Dose 1**	**Dose 2**	**Dose 3**
<48h	0.2	0.1	0.1
2-7d	0.2	0.2	0.2
>7d	0.2	0.25	0.25

Give q12-24h IV over 20-30 min. Check serum creatinine and urine output prior to each dose.

5. **Diagnostic Considerations:** ABG, chest X-ray, ECG, CBC, electrolytes.

FORMULAS

Normal urine output = 50 ml/kg/d
Oliguria = 0.5 ml/kg/h
Normal feedings = 5 oz/kg/d
Formula = 20 calories/ounce, 24 cal/oz, 27 cal/oz
Ounce = 30 cc
Caloric Needs = 100 cal/kg/d
Calories/Kg = cc of formula x 30 cc/oz x 20 calories/oz divided by weight.

Weight in Kg = pounds divided by 2.2

Weight in Kg = [age in years x 2] +10

Blood volume (ml) = 80 ml/kg x weight (kg)

Blood Products:

> 10 cc/kg RBC will raise Hct 5%
> 0.1 unit/kg platelets will raise platelet count, 25000/mm3.
> 1 U/kg of Factor VIII will raise level by 2%.

A-a gradient = $[(P_B-PH_2O) FiO_2 - PCO_2/R] - PO_2$ arterial

P_B = 760 mm Hg PH_2O = 47 mm Hg   R = 0.8 NL <10-15 mm Hg

Arterial oxygen capacity=Hgb(gm)/100 ml x 1.36 ml O2/gm Hgb

Arterial O2 content = 1.36(Hgb)(SaO2)+0.003(PaO2)=NL 20 vol%

O2 delivery = CO x arterial O2 content=NL 640-1000 ml O2/min

Cardiac output = HR x stroke volume

$$CO \text{ L/min} = \frac{125 \text{ ml O2/min/M}^2}{8.5 \{(1.36)(Hgb)(SaO2) (1.36)(Hgb)(SvO2)\}} \times 100$$

$$SVR = \frac{MAP - CVP}{CO_{L/min}} \times 80 = NL \ 800\text{-}1200 \text{ dyne/sec/cm}^2$$

$$PVR = \frac{PA - PCWP}{CO_{L/min}} \times 80 = NL \ 45\text{-}120 \text{ dyne/sec/cm}^2$$

Anion Gap = Na + K - (Cl + HCO3)

$$\text{Adult GFR} = \frac{(140 - age) \ x \ wt \ in \ Kg}{72 \ (males) \ x \ serum \ Cr}$$
$$85 \ (females) \ x \ serum \ Cr$$

$$\text{Cr clearance} = \frac{\text{U Cr (mg/100 mL)} \times \text{U vol (mL)}}{\text{P Cr (mg/100 mL)} \times \text{time (1440 min for 24h)}}$$

Adult Normal Cr clearance =   100-125 ml/min (males),
                              85-105 (females)

$$\text{Body water deficit (L)} = \frac{0.6(\text{weight kg})([\text{Na serum}]-140)}{140}$$

$$\text{Osmolality} = 2[\text{Na} + \text{K}] + \frac{\text{BUN}}{2.8} + \frac{\text{glucose}}{18} = \text{NL 270-290 mOsm/kg}$$

$$\text{Fractional excreted Na} = \frac{\text{U Na/ Serum Na}}{\text{U Cr/ Serum Cr}} \times 100 = \text{NL}<1\%$$

$$\begin{array}{l}\text{Corrected} = \text{measured Na} + \frac{\text{serum glucose (mg/dl)}}{36} = \text{NL 140 mEq/L} \\ \text{serum Na+}\end{array}$$

Corrected = measured Ca + 0.8 x (4 - albumin)
serum Ca+

Basal energy expenditure (BEE):
  Males = 66 + (13.7 x actual weight in Kg) + (5 x height in cm) - (6.8 x age)
  Females = 655 + (9.6 x actual weight in Kg) + (1.7 x height in cm) - (4.7 x age)

Nitrogen Balance = Gm protein intake/6.25 - urine urea nitrogen - (3-4 gm/d
                              insensible loss)

ORDER FORM

Books and Software from Current Clinical Strategies Publishing:

Current Clinical Strategies, Practice Parameters for Medicine, Primary Care, Family Practice, and Gynecology	#___ x $16.75
Current Clinical Strategies, **PEDIATRIC** PHYSICIAN'S DRUG RESOURCE	#___ x $8.75
Handbook of Anesthesiology Mark Ezekiel, MD	#___ x $8.75
Manual of HIV/AIDS Therapy Laurence Peiperl, MD	#___ x $8.75
Current Clinical Strategies, MEDICINE, Paul D. Chan, MD NEW 1994 edition	#___ x $8.75
Current Clinical Strategies, GYNECOLOGY & OBSTETRICS, NEW 1995 edition	#___ x $10.75
Current Clinical Strategies, PEDIATRICS, NEW 1994 edition	#___ x $8.75
FAMILY MEDICINE, NEW 1995 edition Pediatrics, Medicine, Gynecology, Obstetrics	#___ x $26.25
DIAGNOSTIC HISTORY & PHYSICAL EXAMINATION in MEDICINE	#___ x $8.75
OUTPATIENT MEDICINE	#___ x $8.75
CRITICAL CARE MEDICINE	#___ x $12.75
PSYCHIATRY	#___ x $8.75
HANDBOOK OF PSYCHIATRIC DRUG THERAPY	#___ x $8.75
Current Clinical Strategies, SURGERY	#___ x$8.75
Current Clinical Strategies, PHYSICIAN'S DRUG RESOURCE (Adult dosages)	#___ x $8.75

**Current Clinical Strategies, Prescription Writer
Computer Program
Prescription Writing System & Record Manager for MS
Windows.** Produces legible prescriptions in seconds, and keeps
an updated list of each patient's medications.   Includes a
database of over 1500 dosages. PC computer and MS Windows
required; dot matrix or laser printer.   Uses plain paper or Rx
paper (included). **Available 4/30/95**.
Please circle one: 5¼   3½ inch diskettes   #___ x $55.00

Shipping and Handling, add $2.00 per book $ _____

Total $ _____

Enclose the cover of your old edition, and receive $2.00 off your order when you purchase the
new edition.

Please complete reverse side.

Prices are in US dollars. Other countries, send equivalent amount in foreign check. Prices and availability subject to change without notice.

Order by Phone: 714-965-9400 (add $1.50 COD charge per order; a bill will be sent with order)

Order by Mail. Send order & check payable to:

Current Clinical Strategies Publishing
9550 Warner Ave, Suite 213
Fountain Valley, Ca USA 92708-2822

Return Address: _____

_____

_____

_____

Phone Number: (_____)_____

Is this book sold at your local medical book store? ___ yes ___ no
Name of bookstore that does not carry our books:

_____

_____

_____

Comments:

We appreciate your comments about our books and software. Suggested additions, problems or criticisms:

_____

_____

_____

_____

_____

_____

_____

_____

_____

ORDER FORM

Books and Software from Current Clinical Strategies Publishing:

Current Clinical Strategies, Practice Parameters for Medicine, Primary Care, Family Practice, and Gynecology	#___ x $16.75
Current Clinical Strategies, **PEDIATRIC** PHYSICIAN'S DRUG RESOURCE	#___ x $8.75
Handbook of Anesthesiology Mark Ezekiel, MD	#___ x $8.75
Manual of HIV/AIDS Therapy Laurence Peiperl, MD	#___ x $8.75
Current Clinical Strategies, MEDICINE, Paul D. Chan, MD NEW 1994 edition	#___ x $8.75
Current Clinical Strategies, GYNECOLOGY & OBSTETRICS, NEW 1995 edition	#___ x $10.75
Current Clinical Strategies, PEDIATRICS, NEW 1994 edition	#___ x $8.75
FAMILY MEDICINE, NEW 1995 edition Pediatrics, Medicine, Gynecology, Obstetrics	#___ x $26.25
DIAGNOSTIC HISTORY & PHYSICAL EXAMINATION in MEDICINE	#___ x $8.75
OUTPATIENT MEDICINE	#___ x $8.75
CRITICAL CARE MEDICINE	#___ x $12.75
PSYCHIATRY	#___ x $8.75
HANDBOOK OF PSYCHIATRIC DRUG THERAPY	#___ x $8.75
Current Clinical Strategies, SURGERY	#___ x$8.75
Current Clinical Strategies, PHYSICIAN'S DRUG RESOURCE (Adult dosages)	#___ x $8.75

Current Clinical Strategies, Prescription Writer Computer Program

Prescription Writing System & Record Manager for MS Windows. Produces legible prescriptions in seconds, and keeps an updated list of each patient's medications. Includes a database of over 1500 dosages. PC computer and MS Windows required; dot matrix or laser printer. Uses plain paper or Rx paper (included). **Available 4/30/95.**
Please circle one: 5¼   3½ inch diskettes   #___ x $55.00

Shipping and Handling, add $2.00 per book	$ _____
Total	$ _____

Enclose the cover of your old edition, and receive $2.00 off your order when you purchase the new edition.

Please complete reverse side.

Prices are in US dollars. Other countries, send equivalent amount in foreign check. Prices and availability subject to change without notice.

Order by Phone: 714-965-9400 (add $1.50 COD charge per order; a bill will be sent with order)

Order by Mail. Send order & check payable to:

Current Clinical Strategies Publishing
9550 Warner Ave, Suite 213
Fountain Valley, Ca USA 92708-2822

Return Address: _____

_____

_____

_____

Phone Number: (_____)_____

Is this book sold at your local medical book store? ___ yes ___ no
Name of bookstore that does not carry our books:

_____

_____

_____

Comments:

We appreciate your comments about our books and software.

Suggested additions, problems or criticisms:

_____

_____

_____

_____

_____

_____

_____

_____

_____

_____